Sex Education

Published by :
Lotus Press Publishers & Distributors

Sex Education

Dr. Rajeev Sharma
M.D., D.Lit.

Lotus Press
4735/22, Prakash Deep Building
Ansari Road, Darya Ganj,
New Delhi - 110002

Lotus Press Publishers & Distributors
Unit No. 220, 2nd Floor, 4735/22, Prakash Deep Building,
Ansari Road, Darya Ganj, New Delhi-110002
Ph.: 23280047, 41325510, 98118-38000
• E-mail : lotuspress1984@gmail.com
www.lotuspress.co.in

Sex Education

ISBN: 81-8382-064-6

Attention Readers:

Every effort is made to ensures accuracy of material, but the publisher, printer and author will not be held responsible for any inadvertent error(s). In case of any dispute, all legal matters to be settled under Delhi Jurisdiction only.

Printed & Published by : **Lotus Press Publishers & Distributors,** New Delhi-02

Preface

Sex is an act which provides us pleasure and enjoyment. If it is performed between mature and married couples, then it's charm increases to new heights and there is no guilte feeling.

This book is an effort to educate youngesters to educate them about anatomy and physiology of sex organs, how to achieve orgasm, impotency and frigidity, medicines, and all you wanted to know about sex. The book also includes with a separate chapter in the form of questions and answers, in which, most of your querries will be answered.

If you have any querries, you can write to me with a reply envelop, but please do not come without taking prior appointment on phone.

With thanks & regards,

Dr. Rajeev Sharma
Srijan - Aarogya Jyoti®
Palm - 11/03, Shipra Sun City
Indirapuram, Ghaziabad (U.P.)
Ph. : 0120-3020206
email : sharmarajeev108@ rediffmail.com
drrajeev@newkamastura.com

A Brief About Dr. Rajeev Sharma

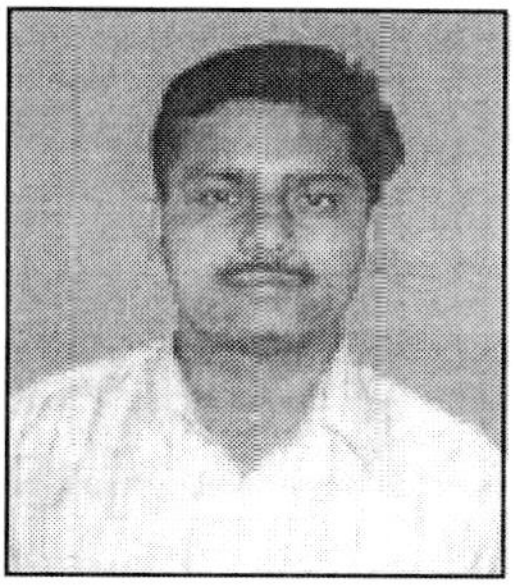

Dr. Rajeev Sharma is an eminent consultant of Homoeopathy,Yoga, Naturopathy and Alternative Medicine in India. He has written more than 200 books in Hindi and English and around 1500 articles, which have been published in various newspapers and magazines. He is also a member of the Editiorial Board of the prestigious *Asian Homoeopathic Journal* besides many other newspapers and magazines.

Dr. Rajeev Sharma has written books on ayurveda, homoeopathy, yoga, naturopahty, accupressure, magnetotherapy, water-therapy, massage and aromatherapy, etc.

He has written books on all major ailments like diabetes, hypertension, obesity, stomach and respiratory disorders, E.N.T. disorders, female and male disorders, UTI disorder, sexual disorders, paediatric problems, headache, stress and other mental problems, etc.

The books written by Dr. Rajeev Sharma have been published by renowned publishers of India like :- Pustak Mahal (Publisher of *Rapidex English Speaking Course*), Diamond Pocket Books (Publisher of Osho literature, *Greha Laxmi, Cricket Today* and *Sadhna Path*), B. Jain Publisher (largest publisher of book on homoeopathy and alternative medicine in India). Jaypee Brothers Medical Publishers, Crest Publishing House, and Manoj Publications.

Dr. Rajeev Sharma is Medical Advisor to Ralson Remedies (a homoeopathic medicine manufacturer), and Dixit Pharmacy (Ayurvedic Medicine Manufacturer), Medical Examiner at the Life Insurance Corporation of India and M.O. in U.P. Govt. He has received several prizes for his outstanding achievements. He has been awarded the *Best Author prize in Hindi* by the Home Ministry and Ministry of Health and Family Welfare, Government of India and *Sarjana Puraskar* by U.P. Hindi Sansthan, Lucknow. He has delivered talks on All India Radio and lectures on Alternative Medicine in various Government and Non-government Organisations. He has written Advertising scripts for the products of several companies.

Dr. Rajeev Sharma is also a social activist. He has worked a lot against Drug Abuse and prevention of AIDS. Now-a-days, he is working on a project to check the population growth of India with an NGO called 'Nav Chetna Manch'. He has worked for pollution control and human rights too and has received the World Human Rights Promotion Award. His name has been published in *LIMCA BOOK OF RECORDS 2005*. He has developed two websites too — www.newkamasutra.com; and www.indiaalive.net

Contents

The Human Sex Organs

Male Sex Organs

The sex organs of a male are quite complicated form of a reproductive system. They produce semen, store it and release it into the woman's vagina at the time of ejaculation. The procreation, therefore, is the result of the union of the sperm cell and the ovum.

The Testes

The male organs comprises of the two testes or testicles hung side by side in a sac called the scrotum, behind the penis in its relaxed state. The testes, oval in shape and about an inch long and an inch wide, have two different functions. These are made up of a series of jobs composed of minute tubules in which the sperm cells, the spermatozoa, are formed and liberated. The internal secretion of sex harmones, which create sex impulse and cause the essential male characteristics in the individual and play its role with the other secretion glands in the body in sustaining the normal functioning of the body, are achieved by it. In case this function is impaired before puberty, the development of the individual becomes seriously altered in form, temperament and impulses, Since it is directly absorbed into the blood, these secretions are termed as internal secretion.

In the seminal discharge the male sperms formed in the testes are the vital elements because these sperms have the power of fertilising the egg of the woman to conceive a new life. These highly vitalized cells consist of a head, neck and long tail. It is in this head the nucleus is contained which transmit the hereditary characteristics of the individual. Having the power of independent motion, these sperms propel themselves in the liquid secretion in which it floats its tails having a float-rate approximately its own length per second. After the semen's discharge, it requires an hour or more for the sperms to reach the tube where it fertilises an ovum (egg.). When the released female egg encounters one male sperm or spermatozoa, it penetrates the cell wall of the egg in a complex series of rearrangement of the elements of both cells, known as fertilization . Through in a single male orgasm about 200 to 500 million sperms are discharged, only one is able to reach the walls of the cell. The remaining sperms are cast out along with the other residues of the physiological process. The spermatozoa are being slowly formed and released in the testicles all the time.

The Epididymis and vas Deferens : Each of the cluster of convoluted tubes in the lobes of the testes, in which the sperm cells are formed, merges into a single tube, and the resulting mass of tubes in turn forms a complex network which constitutes a large annex to the body of the testes. It is known as epididyms. The network of tubes of the epididyms unite in turn to form the seminal duct or vas deferens. From the epididyms each seminal duct upwards in the scrotalm sac and enters the pelvis cavity where it continues its upward course, then curves forward and downward to enter the Urethra which contains the urine from the bladder.

The Seminal Vesicles

The vas, two in number, issuing from each testes take a round of the bladder and then empty into seminal vesicles. These vesicles are two small pouches, situated just behind the urinary bladder. The function of seminal vesicles is to store the semen and secrete a gelatinous substance which by mixing with the sperm thickens the semen and increases it volume. The secretion also provides nourishment and strength to sperms.

Since these testes and seminal vesicles are always secreting and manufacturing semen, sometimes the vesicles are filled to capacity and the nature empties them in the form of nocturnal emissions as is in the process of orgasm. The phenomenon is usually accompanied by an erotic dream and the pleasurable sex feelings of an orgasm.

It is a mistaken belief of old Indian theories that nocturnal emissions or wet dream are sign of weakness. These are natural, harmless occurrences to be expected in most normal men, particularly between the ages of fourteen and thirty five. There is nothing to worry about. Untold mental torture and unnecessary expenses has been caused to millions of men through the miser presentation of quacks who prey upon the ignorance and fear of men in these matters.

Seminal emissions vary greatly in frequency between different men and in the same man at different times. Within the normal men, the frequency may range between once a month to several times a week. Many factors—physical, mental, and temperamental—are responsible for it. There are some young men who rarely or never experience nocturnal emissions. Though the occurrence of emissions are natural, there absence does not necessarily indicate any abnormality. It is quite possible in their case that the contents naturally ooze out in the ducts, aided by bowel movements to be thrown out with urine from the bladder.

Nocturnal emission generally occur when a man sleeps on his back. The reason being that in the position the weight of the partly filled or full bladder resting upon the vesicles increases the irritation to set off the reflexes ejaculating semen. To avoid this, heavy food should not be taken before going to bed and constipation should not be allowed.

The Prostate Gland

It is shaped like a horse chest. Surrounding the neck of the bladder and the junction of the urinary and spermatic ducts, into which juncture the prostate empties its contents through some thirty outlets. The prostate secretion is also added to the semen before it is ejaculated in the vagina. Thus semen is combined product of all these glands. Each of these glands imparts to the semen its many peculiar characteristics. The prostate is also a sexual gland which is situated below the urinary bladder. During coital climax, the prostate contracts and mixes its own secretion in the semen. To sustain sexual vigour and strength, it is considered necessary that the prostate functions properly. The prostate secretes a thin, milky alkaline fluid, the function of which is similar to the ducts of the vesicles. The alkalinity serves to protect the spermatozoa against acidity arising from the urine. This acidity damages the vitality of the sperm cells.

The Urethra

A small duct called urethra runs through the centre of the penis down to its glands from the urinary bladder. This duct serves the double purpose—it empties urine from the bladder and ejaculates the semen from seminal vesicles. Thus urethra is intimately connected with both the systems of seminal discharge and urine elimination. The urethra in penis discharges both semen and urine but sex mechanism of male body is such that both the actions cannot take place together . During seminal discharge a special valve automatically shuts off the urine.

The Penis

A child's penis is small in size which grows long with the other organs of the body after the onset of puberty. The penis, through which the bladder is emptied and the sperm discharged during intercourse, is normally three to four inches long and in normal flaccid state about one and a quarter to two inches in diameter. When a man is sexually aroused his penis grows erect, the organ measures about one and half inches in diameters and five and a half to six inches in length along its upper side. It is made up in part of spongy tissue which becomes gorged with blood, making the organ hard and rigid. The erection is necessary in order to achieve the penetration of the vagina. In response to mechanical or psychological, i.e. stimulation, the erection is achieved through a nervous mechanism which causes a rush of blood into the organ and at the same time greatly restricts its flow, thus causing rigid distension of the penis. Like the size the shape also varies from man to man. Penis is the male organ which releoses the semen into vagina. There is no correlation between the size of a penis and man's sexual strength and capacity. The erect size also does not make much difference because the vagina has such an elastic cavity to accommodate any size of the penis. The most sensitive nerve ending in a vagina is the clitoris which can always be reached by any penis howsoever it be small.

The Glans Penis

The foremost end of the penis round like a knob, is called glans penis. It is slightly thicker than the rest of the shaft. In the flaccid state of the penis the head or glans penis is partly or wholly covered by a loose layer of the skin, in the uncircumcised men, called the prepuce or foreskin. This is retracted for the purpose of cleaning and it becomes naturally retracted after entry in coitus. The surface of the foreskin is somewhat mucus owing to the gland which secrete a substance called smegma. It is an irritating secretion and should be regularly cleaned, otherwise it makes the forepart of the penis to become cheesy in appearance by breeding germs. It should be washed daily with soap. The glans penis has the most sensitive nerve endings. A slight soft touch to excite a man and to make the penis erect. It is the mainly the penis on which a little rubbing whether by hand or vaginal contact sends the sex waves in the entire body, culminating, in orgasm or ejaculation.

The Erection and Ejaculation

As also referred to earlier, the effect of the sexual arousal in man is physical manifestation in the erection of the penis. A direct and gentle stimulation of penis almost always causes erection. This is borne out of a relax action and may occur in sleep. Erection may be caused without any rubbing of the penis just by erotic thoughts even. In the early morning it may be aroused because of the urge to urinate. Most such erections terminate without any discharge.

Ejaculation is the culmination of sexual stimulation in man. Having entered the vagina, the most sensitive nerve endings of which the penis is made up, become tense and excited on account of the friction against the walls of vagina, it may experience further fanned by the secretion of fluids in the vagina. To and fro movements of the penis add on the arousal. The tension gets higher and higher till it reaches the climax to explode and get released. This process of the climax and the release of the seminal fluids is known as ejaculation. The basic difference between the sex mechanism of man and woman is that in the man climax and ejaculation or orgasm take place simultaneously while in woman these are two different states. At the time of climatic height and orgasm the seminal discharge takes place through the penis in number of spurts. The number of the spurt varies from 4 to 20 Just as the first menses indicates the onset of puberty in a girl, in a boy the first ejaculation marks the entrance into adolescence.

Female Organs

The female organs are more complicated. They are confined in the body and not openly visible. Because of their apparent invisibility, Indian girls are ignorant about their organs. Hence it is more necessary that full knowledge about the female organs structure and their functions be discussed in full detail.

The Vulva

The two visibly fleshy folds, covered with hair are the outer lips or labia Majora. When parted they reveal two smaller or inner lips or labia. The insides of the inner are covered with the mucous membranes. The inner lips of labia are one of the several sexual sensation centres. During sexual intercourse these labia remain constantly massaged by the rubbing of the penis. In some women the inner lips protrude somewhat. The inner lips meet at their upper ends which when separated look like the form of the wishbone of a hen.

The principal organ of the sex feeling, the clitoris, is situated just above junction of the inner lips. The clitoris looks like a mini penis having erectile tissue and a head and free skin similar to the penis of the man. it is covered from above by a hood of skin. The clitoris is made of highly sensitive nerves which respond very well to sexual stimulation. It is from this centre that the sexual feeling begins and permeates in the entire body through vulva and vagina. When erect, the clitoris looks like the size or shape of a small bean. About an inch below the clitoris is a small opening of the tube called urethra. Its duct conducts the urine from the bladder. The urethra has only the urinary function and no sexual function.

The mucous membrane above the clitoris, like the penis of the man, is covered with glands which secret smegma. Owing to the structure, cleanliness in the woman is a little more difficult than in the man.

It is not only hygienically necessary to keep it clean but also for this reason that it emits foul smell which tend to inhibit sexual desire in the man.

The Hymen

Just below the urinary passage is the entrance to vagina. In a normal virgin girl, this opening remains partially closed by a thin membrane called the hymen. Though it appears in different shapes but normally it looks like a crescent in shape appearing like the forward extension of the black walls of the vagina. In many cases during the first intercourse when the hymen is ruptured there may be slight bleeding and pain. It is a false notion that the hymen is the symbol of virginity. A nicked or stretched or tattered hymen does not mean the body has been penetrated into. It could be ruptured on account of jerks or falls that a young girl might experience. Many girls may not have much of it or others may lose it in doing some kind of vigorous job. Sometimes the insertion of a finger into the vagina may prove too hard for any hymen. Occasionally a hymen is so tough that it remain intact even after several sessions of sexual intercourse. It all depends on the kind of hymen a girl is born with. Generally during the first coitus, the penis tears it in several places by its thrust. Repeated sexual intercourse continue to tear it till hardly a few shreds mark its former presence. At times, in certain cases, it was found to be so flexible that instead of breaking into pieces by the penile thrust, it merely bends and allows the penis to gild over it. In some cases the surgeon's aid is obtained to slit open the membranes. But the bleeding and discomfort, when they occur, are not of sufficient consequence to warrant fear on the part of the woman. Therefore, it is important that fear be eliminated and that the woman enter into the first coitus with gay abandon. This is psychologically important because this fear powerfully inhibits her sexual responses and the function of the lubricating glands, leaving the parts dry. This increases the probability of discomfort and bleeding and diminishes the possibility of experiencing any sexual pleasure at the first coitus.

The Vagina

It is a tube or canal extending from vulva to the neck of the uterus. It is three and half (3½) to 4 inches in length in its normal relaxed position. It is here that the penis in intercourse is sheathed with its elastic walls. It receives the seminal discharge and allows the sperm to travel forward towards the womb in search of an ovum. It is through this tube that a child passes to the outside world. During pregnancy, the vagina and its outlet becomes capable of great expansion permitting the passage of the child from the womb without injury in may cases. In most instances, however, more or less laceration of the muscular structure controlling the opening of the vagina may occur. It should be vitally important that such tears receive prompt surgical attention. The use and control of the muscles about the vaginal opening and of the entire pelvic floor are necessary to the woman's most effective participation in coitus. The relaxed condition and the loss of muscular control which results from the failure to repair perennial and vaginal tears may result in greatly diminishing sexual satisfaction in coitus for both partners, and may render it impossible for the woman to achieve orgasm at all. The flexible walls of the vagina are lined by a mucous membrane secreting a fine fluid which keeps it moist and clean. It has great releasing and contracting power. It is because of this reason that the vagina besides being made up of flexible walls, is able to accommodate much larger penis not withstanding its small cavity.

The Womb or Uterus

It is pear shaped organ of heavy muscular walls. The virgin uterus measures about two to three quarters of inches in length and two inches wide. Its elastic muscles expand considerably during pregnancy with the growth of the baby. Its upper part is connected with ovaries by two ducts called fallopian tubes. The organ is supported in the pelvis by strong ligaments. Its position is at right angles to the vagina, the upper, heavy end being directed forward towards the front of the pelvis. The small end (cervix) opens into the vagina and closes its upper end. After childbirth, the organ gradually retracts to its former size. The organ has powerful muscles to help push the baby out through vagina. During pregnancy the uterus retains and supplies nourishment to the growing baby till the delivery.

The Fallopian Tubes and Ovaries

The upper end of the uterus, as referred earlier, are joined by the fallopian tubes each about five and a half inches long, which extend right and left to the ovaries. The function of the fallopian tube is to conduct ovum from the ovaries to the uterus. This is achieved through contractile action of the tubes finger like fringes called fimbria. The sweeping motion of fimbria is in one direction, which helps egg cells in moving towards uterus. In most cases, the fertilization of an egg cell or ovum takes place during its journey through the fallopian tube. The process of passing of an egg cell through the tube is called ovulation. The fertilised egg is then moved down the tube towards the womb.

The ovaries are alike to the testes of the male. They produce the female reproductive cells, the Ova or eggs, and internal secretions. Situated at the outer ends of the tubes, one on each side of the uterus, an ovary is about the size and shape of a large almond in the shell. Though they are comparable to the testes in their function, the hormone function of the ovaries is apparently more complete than that of the testes of the male. In addition to the internal secretion which governs the development of the specific female character and help to sustain the normal functioning of the individual as an organism, the ovaries elaborate other chemical substances which control the reproductive functions. Just like the castration performed on male, if the ovaries are removed before puberty the development of the individual get will drastically altered.

When a girl is born, her ovaries already contain these egg cells of ova in thousands. But then these are not mature. With the onset of puberty the ovaries start their work of maturing ovum. During the life time of woman about 400-500 of egg cells mature. From the time of puberty till menopause, every month a mature egg is produced by one of the ovaries. The mature egg cells passes through the fallopian tube towards the uterus. If an egg is fertilised it starts growing before it enters the velventry lined uterus which nourishes the egg, it remains alive for about 20-24 hours after entering the tube and then it disintegrates and gets absorbed into the body.

The Menstruation

When the egg cell is not fertilized, the monthly preparation by the womb to receive a fertilized egg cell goes a waste and the debris is cast out - the whole process is known as menstruation. Mesntruation generally continues for three to five days but even longer in few cases. While it is a normal physiological function, not to be regarded as sickness or being unwell, in severe cases the general let down and the readjustments of the entire organism do involve nervous tensions and in many cases a variety of aches and pains for which due allowance is to be made in the social and personal circle of the individual. It should be clearly understood that a girl or woman, during this period should not be considered an untouchable as she is in most of the communities in India. As a matter of fact, the underlying reason of this belief was sympathetic, that in a period of menstruation, a girl or a lady might feel weak so she should be given full rest which was mistakenly converted into a hygienic one. But now-a-days no educated girl or woman adhere to these obscurantic norms and treat the period day like any other day in their life. May be because of better facilities to contain this blood into the sanitary napkins, the modern woman does not make it a show of it. It is not physically but emotionally a woman might feel disturbed during this period.

The Breasts

Though the breasts do not strictly come under the categories of the organs we are discussing, they are being induced because of their especial significance in manifestation of the sexual arousal of a woman. Specially their breast nipples signify as one of the most sensitive erogenous zones on a woman's body. Squeezing, sucking, caressing of the breasts, particularly the nipples give rise to strong and most favourable sexual desires. The sexologists feel that in the initial stages of married life, a woman drives more pleasure from any such stimulation of her breast than the actual coitus. Nipples like clitoris have erectile tissues and very sensitive nerves endings. These tissues become firm and erect during erotic stimulation. It is for this reason that breasts or mammary glands are two very important sexual organs, whole development is dependent on the secretion of certain harmones of the female sex. Though the breasts have their primary function in feeding a newborn child, their importance as a neurotic and sensitive zone permeating with desire to mate has great significance in sexual relationship. Although their sizes vary from puberty to maturity and they grow large during pregnancy, the sexual undertones of this organise have influenced. An ideally formed breast has always been the most beautiful female symbol or characteristic.

Difference Between Men and Women

From incidence of heart disease to tolerance of pain to strategies for seduction, men and women go their separate ways. Here are some facts to prove it.

Body talk - The average adult Indian Male is 5-foot-8; the average female, 5-foot-2. He carries1½ times as much muscle as she does, and half as much fat.

High hopes - Men tack on an average of more than half an inch to their true height, while women subtract more than two pounds from their true weight, according to the Metropolitan Insurance Company.

The longevity gap - In the United States, women live 665 days long than men. At age 65, the ratio of surviving women to men is 100 to 65. Hang around. Gerontologist Seven Fox, D.O., says, "By following a healthy exercise regimen alone, men could increase their longevity by about 9 percent."

Yeah, but what if Sex magazine had done the survey ? For men, money and sex are equally important, but for women, money is on their mind more often than sex, accordion to a survey by Money magazine. And more women said they enjoy money more than sex, according to a survey by Money magazine.

Tab hunters - More women than men take vitamins. An estimated 88 million women use vitamin and mineral products, compared with 81 million men.

The burden of proof. More than 8 percent of men are alcoholics, compared with only 3.5 percent of women, according to the National Institute on Alcohol Abuse and Alcoholism. Men can drink more than women before suffering health problems because their metabolism of alcohol is faster.

"Not tonight, dear...." - Men suffer fewer aches and pains than women, reports USA Today. Women feel at least one symptom of discomfort (headache, fatigue, etc.) more than 43 percent of the time, compared with men's 28 percent. Then again, men find it twice as tough as women to take the same amount of chronic pain. Being in pain is also more likely to lower a man's self-esteem than a woman's.

Remember the Maine vacation ? Women remember better than men, and the discrepancy increases with age. In a word-recall test at Johns Hopkins Medical Institution, men generally lagged slightly behind women; men in their late sixties scored a full 20 percent lower than did women of the same age.

Eye-opener - Men have a weaker sense of smell than women, but are more sensitive to light.

Joint custody - Males in their senior year of high school are only slightly more likely to have smoked marijuana (63 percent) than are women (56 percent), according to *Drugs in American Society* by Rich Good. However, the boys were more than twice as likely to be daily users - 10 percent versus 4 percent.

No kidding - We all can dish it out, but who can take it ? According to *Psychology Today*, men and women equally resent criticism from their mates, but men take it more to heart when their kids put them down.

Defence mechanism - Men are more likely than women are to favour spendig money on nuclear weapons, according to *Source* magazine. Men also tend to view military defense issues in simpler terms, while women tend to have a more complex perspective.

Look who's talking - Men converse mostly about news

events and work; women talk mostly about food and health, according to a study published in *U.S. News and World Report*.

Wheel difference - Men drive more than twice as many miles as women annually : Men average 13,412 miles; women, 6,079.

Can't touch this - Women are more prone than men to get ripply fat - sometimes called cellulite - on their thighs and buttocks because the fibres holding their skin to muscle are in parallel cords. This structure permits fat to bulge through and marble the skin. You seldom see celulite on men because under the skin men have a dense mesh of fibers, which unites the fat in one smooth layer.

Provide and conquer - Men tend to choose a mate based on good looks. For women, a man's looks are not as important as his social status and wealth, says David Buss, Ph.D., a psychologist at the University of Michigan.

Close calls - Men feel nearly as much need for intimacy as women but experience it differently, according to a study done at Loyola University of Chicago. For women, intimacy leads to more satisfaction in their roles as wife and mother. For men, being able to be close with people creates confidence and resiliency that lets them go out and conquer the world.

Wild thing - Men's preferred home activity is sex, while women's is spending time with the family (number two for men), according to surveys by R.H. Bruskin Market Research and Speiged.

Doctored facts - Men exercise more strenuously than women do, but they also smoke and drink more, finds a study at Pennsylvania State University. Women know more about nutrition, and they get more eye exams and dental and blood pressure check-ups.

Everyone out of the pool - According to a Gallup survey, the most popular sport for men is fishing. Women's most popular sport ? Swimming.

The pits. It may be indelicate to say so, but women's are smellier. Men perspire more heavily on their chests and women more heavily under their arms.

Wake up, Irene - Studies suggest that men spend more time in shallow sleep as they get older and may even start skipping deep sleep altogether, says Arthur Spielman, Ph.D., director of the Insominia Treatment Centre in New York. For unknown reasons, aging doesn't affect women's sleep as much.

Left learning - Most men put their pants on left leg first, while the majority of women start with the right leg.

Eat and run - Men are 31 percent more likely to choose foods and beverages to improve athletic performance but find it more difficult to eat healthful snacks than women, according to a poll by Health Focus, a Pennsylvania food consulting firm.

A man's heart - Men have double the risk of heart disease than women have, a tendency that some researchers attribute to the male hormone, testosteorone. Evidently the hormone triggers the production of cholesterol. Men also have higher blood levels of stress hormones, which cause the heart to beat harder and blood pressure to rise.

Bully for you - A narrowing study found that most school bullies are male, and that while the tendency of boys to bully rose with age, in girls it dropped. Researchers conclude aggression is partly biological in nature and, again, testosterone may be the spur.

Dieting - One out of three women diet, compared with one out of five men.

How to Educate about Sex

There is a misplaced notion that the kids would go the 'wrong way' if they are educated about sex which is an unfounded fear, for the simple reason that unguided youth is more prone and amenable to 'Pitfalls' than a properly guided youth. The child is not aware that fire can burn also but, when he is cautioned in time, he will take safeguards lest he is burnt by leeping flames. Ignorance about sex is far more dangerous than sex guidance. After all, someone has to take up the challenge. Evasion of this sacred duty is frought with dire consequences, much to the detriment of the young ones, though elders cannot escape the onus of being willynilly and evasive.

Following methods may be adopted to educate a child about sex, right from class VIII when physical changes start surfacing, much to the amazement of the young ones.

1. The parents (preferably the mother or elder sister or elder brother's wife) can guide the child as to how changes in body take place' - function of each sex-organ and the risks involved in playing 'mischief' with the organs. The teachers, at school, can, during the course of studies, well upon the subject in a better way to unravel the so-called mysteries and 'secrets' of sex. In my opinion, school is the best forum for such educative devices.
2. Let physiology be a compulsory subject in the school

syllabus, so that more light is thrown upon the subject. When the minds of students are attuned such a way that they are motivated to attend such classes, they will always develop fancy for the subject, since they would also be examined.

3. In the absence of sex-education at school or home, let there be display of audio cassettes which should be followed by video cassettes. Whatever the student has heard and, at a latter stage, when video cassettes are played, he would be able to correlate the Audio and Video versions. At this stage, the teacher should step in and reply to queries of his students and if all the inquisitive queries have been aptly replied to, the students will gain a lot. Let us freely take advantage from the facilities made available by the electronic media.
4. A question-answer session will solve most of the problems, relating to sex education.
5. At the XII standard, functions of sex organs should be explained fully. Here also audio-video cassettes can easily achieve the desired result.
6. Due to certain taboos and social inhibitions, it may be a bit embarrasing for a lady teacher to suitably reply to queries from male students and vice versa. In order to avoid such an awkward situation, let the lady teachers guide, educate and reply to girl students, and male teachers should do the same job for their male students.
7. There is no harm if combined classes, in a coeducational institute, are taken by both male and female teachers
8. Let there be inter-school seminars where teachers, psychiatrists, doctors etc. may take part to dole out their advice and guidance to the young folk. It will provide wider exposure of views, ideas, facts, discussions. Doubts can also be allayed by means of group discussions.

Modern youth, these days, have first-hand knowledge of what they ought not to know or practise but, they remain unsafe due to the risks involved in free sex. Their knowledge, gained through porno, periodicals and magazines, serves to ignite their sexual passions and fantasies and to do practically whatever is revealed through the sex postures, depicted in such magazines, x-rated videos, movies etc. This is not a healthy way to sex education. It is simply a means to free sex where passion rides high, and all other sane and safety measures are neglected.

Young people stealthily read porno, literature which vitiates the mind and forces them to premature sex. Had such misguided youth been properly educated about sex, their craving and intensity to indulge in premarital sex would never have arisen. In young age one should acquire proper sex knowledge but must not indulge in unholy sex acts. Incidence of rapes can be easily attributed to such pseudo and premature knowledge. Virgin Mothers' number is on the rise in our society. Situation in elite class is still worse, where there is no check on anyone and one is free to enjoy sex in whatever way and whichever place one wishes, at whatever price.

Whichever methods is adopted, to educate the youth on sex knowledge, emphasis should always be laid on educative, explicit, motivative process. We have to forewarn the youth about hazards and diseases involved in sexual activity keeping an eye on pursuasive approach. If they are properly and timely forewarned, they will remain forearmed also.

How to Teach Sex Education

- Try to teach sex to your child in a matter-of-fact manner, in the same manner as you would talk about any matter with them.
- Do not sermonise or lecture. Be persuasive and sympathetic and make sure that the child's interest remains sustained and element of curiosity stays on.
- If a child poses any question, during the course of

sex education, that must be replied to allay his doubts and/or misconceptions.

- ☞ Your discussion should not be around disclosure of biological factors alone. It should also include values, emotions, decision-making also, since the young ones value such qualities.
- ☞ As children have canny ability to receive and reject, so don't be afraid if your discussion gets prolonged. But, in doing so, make sure that child's interest remains intact. It is your duty to gauge as to how your child reacts to your discussions about sex.
- ☞ Don't ever spurn aside child's queries. If you are evasive, your child will lose faith in you and, as a result thereof, will act indifferently or may be even inattentive.
- ☞ While telling the young one about sexual organs, use only correct terminology, instead of merely referring to 'Pee-Pee' for penis or "bottom" for vagina.
- ☞ They should be advised, fortified with suitable guidelines, about sex abuse and how to say "No" to an adult.
- ☞ In most of the countries puberty begins even from the tenth year, when physical changes like public hair, erection of clitoris, enlargement of breast and prominence of nipples, menstruation etc. start taking places. So, it is always better to educate the child about sex before the said changes surface. It will take away an element of surprise from child's mind and also save the parent from embarrassment of unpalatable questioning.
- ☞ Electronic media, porno magazines and literature, x-rated films have already enhanced children's knowledge about homosexuality, heterosexuality, prostitution, masturbation, self-abuse or child-abuse, etc. So, such aspects must also be part of a parent's sex education programme.
- ☞ Tell the child what is erection of penis and of clitoris

as also what is masturbation, especially to girls. Also explain how and when venereal diseases, AIDS, HIV problems set in, and also disclose the dangers and socio~sexual impacts. Let there not be any fact withheld. Respond to child's enquiries in a receptive, sympathetic and friendly way, so that they don't feel that they have been landed in an awkward position. Let them stay normal.

☞ If a child asks any question which you wish to avoid, then don't rebuke and say "you are too young to learn and know about such things", or strangulate his curiosity by a modified way flat. Let the child feel comfortable and natural.

☞ If you can't or don't wish to reply to any question, you should frankly say a flat 'No', but show no hesitancy in being frank and straight-forward. You can take help from relevant teacher, friend, counsellor, doctor or even a friend, or else you may ask the young one to contact anyone of the said persons to find reply to the queries.

☞ Have a self appraisal, weigh yourself and put a question to yourself 'Whether you have conveyed what you wanted to or you have withheld any fact.'

☞ Induce and encourage your child to put any question, concerning the subject, to you and, when asked, be simply explicit.

Advantages of Sex Education

☞ It will lay emphasis on behavioural, biological, psychosocial, cultural, clinical aspects.

☞ Complexities of human nature, social order, will also find a way in revelations.

☞ Sexual problems can be prevented by better sex education.

☞ Problems of various diseases could be sovled and the aspirant, being well informed in advance, would himself take care of such impediments.

- ☞ It will help one in choosing a suitable partner, so as to lead a happy family life.
- ☞ Above all, dark clouds will give way to bright sunlight, as there could not ever be a better substitute for proper education

Too Young for Love

What happens when Cupid pairs you with someone your parents don't like? Those who are caught in this dilema tend to take refuge in the romantic idealism of the teenage protagonists of classic love stories like Romeo and Juliet. Relationships sans parents' blessings are always a cup of woes for both the young lovers as well as their moms and dads.

Parental Restrictions

For parents, dealing with their love-stuck chilldren is a tricky challenge. The kids themselves would resist any objections to their perfect love and may even break down emotionally. Nilu sharma, a teacher in a South Delhi based school, recounts an experience with her daughter. "I have a 19-year-old teenage daughter. One day I caught her with this guy while shopping. She had been dating him for almost six months. I was against this for I thought it was too early for her to get involved with anyone. Like most moms, I was worried. But how do I approach the subject to her in a manner that would not be seen as encroaching upon her privacy? I chose my words carefully and told her about my displeasure over her seeing a guy at her age. I also made it clear that I had nothing particular against the boy, but I was just concerned.

I didn't want her to end up making mistakes, which teenagers like her are likely to do."

Some parents take a friendly approach when dealing with teenage Romeos. Vijay Anand, a West-Delhi based architect, who found that his 17 year-old son was having an affair with a girl after reading his e-mails accounts, "Initially, I was furious at the discovery. But later, when I thought about it with a cool mind, I realised that society had become more open and liberal about such teenage activities. Anyway, I asked him, more like a friend than a father, what he honestly felt about the girl. His fears were removed and he was quite forthcoming because of my approach. He justified his underage relationship saying that the girl belonged to a decent family and that they shared lot of interests. It was a delicate situation. I told him I fully understood and accepted how he felt for the girl but told him not to take it seriously for there was the risk of getting depressed when it didn't work out. The trick with dealing teenage romance is to be a friend. They should trust you enough to get close and personal with you. It is also essential for parents to respect their feelings and not get furious."

New Age Love

Teenagers see romantic liaisons with a different point of view, and they think there's nothing wrong in having a relationship with a guy at their age.

"When I met this guy at my friend's party, I fell for him instantly. I told myself 'yeah he is the one for me'. Quite confident of myself on this match, I didn't think twice before telling my mom all about him. I was sure she would understand and support me, as she herself had a love marriage. She listened to me patiently, but told me to forget about the relationship before it becomes serious. Still, I persisted arguing that I was not thinking of a lifelong commitment and just wanted to be with him as I liked him.

And no matter what my mother's objections were, I was determined to go ahead with the guy," says Pooja Mehra, a student of Hindu college.

"Parents just can't understand when you are in love. They dismiss our genuine love as a crush or infatuation," adds Gaurav Mittal, a student of Bhagat Singh. "I have been seeing my girlfriend for the last three years who is also studying in my school. When my parents got to know about it from a school friend of mine, my life became miserable. They won't believe that it is for real. Why would I date anyone for three years if it were an infatuation? I am still seeing my girlfriend against their wishes."

Both sides may have their own point of view, but given that the primary motivation is concern for each other, perhaps, the best way is to remember that and look for a middle path.

Unveil Your Romantic Side

Relationships are like little glaciers; under various pressures, they're always moving and changing, gathering all sorts of debris. But after some time, they move so slowly, it's easy to forget they're there, particularly when you live together. To use a more familiar metaphor, one day your relationship is a wild ride, all loops and cork screws, and then, out of nowhere, it's mellowed and straightened out. Actually, it's worse than that. It's stagnating.

With all that in mind, the home you share with your partner presents a bunch of romantic opportunities to reignite that stagnating relationship. The following suggestions, centred around the element of surprise, should get you started:

Give your partner a massage

Your partner comes home from a horrendous day at work, exhausted and even a little bad-tempered. So what do you do? Offer to give a massage. Using aromatherapy oils, focus on their neck and back, the areas that tend to tense up under stress and cause aches and pains. You can create the mood by dimming the lights and lighting candles.

Bring breakfast in bed

A classic gesture, breakfast in bed is the proverial "oldie but goodie." Get up early on a Saturday or Sunday morning and prepare breakfast just the way your partner likes it, with toast, fresh fruit, tea, idlis or whatever. Then surprise them by serving it in bed. Another great way to start the day.

Write romantic notes

The love letter or love note is an amazing thing; litte effort is required to write your partner one, and yet you can express so much. So wirte them a few creative, unique love notes and leave them in unexpected places around the house.

Order In

Order in for dinner and have it waiting for your partner when he gets home. Create a romantic setting by recreating a restaurent feel on the dining room table or in the balcony, complete with plates, silverware and cloth napkins. For an extra romantic touch, add candles and a small vase with some flowers.

Enjoy the cool winters

In the winter, get a fire going on your rooftop (if your society gives you the access). Then, set up some pillows and blankets, and uncork a bottle of wine. If you want to take things to the next level, have a romantic dinner sitting.

Go for a Sauna Bath

The bath tub or a shower is one of the most romantic household locales. Ensure that it is clean, than draw them a hot bath and place aroma oils, lufa, and other exotic bath accessories in the bathroom for your partner to discover.

Alarm Bells.........and how you can help it

There's no sex

Solution : Think of the things that made you attractive to each other once. Have they changed? Have you put on too much weight? Do you never get the time to make love? Address all the micro issues and then go on to bigger problems.

Every time they do something for you, you think of all that you've done for them and make lists

Solution : Maybe you're giving too much in the relationship. While selfless love seems perfect at first, it's not always the best thing. Start giving slightly less to the other person and more to yourself.

With other people you're happy, with your partner you feel flat

Solution : Take time away from the world. Go back to the places you frequented while you were dating, relive those times.

Even when your partner does something nice, you remember all the bad things they've done in the past

Solution : Learn to let go of resentment. Write a letter to your partner. Put down all that makes you angry, sad, afraid, what you regret, what you want and what you appreciate in them. Re-read the letter. Don't send it.

Every time you talk about each other to friends, you end up complaining

Solution : Consciously choose to take more time to talk about the good things in your partner. Make this a habit. While with each other, be gentle about what you dislike. Don't always be gunning for a flight.

Proper Place/Dress/Sounds/ Lights to Enjoy Sex

If you wish to enjoy coitus completely do at least the following preliminaries :

Place

The room where you intend to have coitus should be free from noise, interference and it should be neat, clean, airy, well-ventilated. The collors of bed sheets, curtains, wall paints should conform to personal preference and tastes. Red colour is said to ignite sensuality. Dull, drab, colours should find no place in your sleeping room. Colours play an important part on the mind. Avoid dark red, blue, green and violent colours, as far as possible. Pink cream, fawn colours add to sex pleasure.

Dress

Keeping in view your mood, approach, preference and likes and dislikes of your partner, wear only those clothes which are neither too loose or too tight, rather those should be comfortable, revealing, transparent and sexy. Dress holds a unique place in sex act. Don't put on any dress which is likely to stand in the way of your body handling. Certain couples prefer to wear dresses which expose the bodies, some wish to wear scant clothes or only underwears. Those who wish to resort to strip-tease method should wear only such dresses which can be removed slowly, making way for gradual removal thereof. Some couples prefer to enter in sex in a total nude form.

Colour of dresses should be able to heighten your sexual lust.

Personal Hygiene and Bath

It is necessary that a bath with scented water or using cologne, rose water will do away with foul smell from the body. Bad odour is most likely to drive you away from conjugal love, as most people can't withstand foul body odour, which is an impediment in a turn on. While bathing, take care to wash your mouth, ears, armpits, thigh joints, and genitals thoroughly to ensure proper hygiene. Shave the armpits and hair on the pubic region, on and around genitals and use some pleasing, scented and 'Mild cream and lotion to rule out any chance of infections. When private parts are shaved, creamed/sprayed with lotion, one should experience added flavour in sex, as clean and shaven parts help in an early turn-on.

Spray your neck, ears, ear lobes, armpits, chest, navel portion with scented sprays but the odour of scents used should be pleasing.

Hair should be dressed and combed in such a way that your partner's choice therefore should be quite visibly felt and noticed. Some persons fondle with their partner's hair with gay abandon. Dark, lengthy, curly hair are preferred by most men. If possible, wash your head with same fragrant soap so that the pleasing smell stays for a longer period; at least before, during and after coitus.

Breasts hold an important part in sex arousal. Clean the teats and areola thoroughly so that when your partner sucks, kisses the nipples, no bad taste enters into his mouth,

Under portion of skin folds of breasts should be cleaned properly. Some males hate to see hair on nipples or / and areola. So, if there is any hair thereon, pluck the same. Nipple-sucking is a pleasant and cheerfu exercise.

Use of Lubricants

There should be no aversion and hesitation in applying some cream, oil or any other lubricant to penis, glans of penis, vulva and vagina but it must be ensured that suct lubricants are non-allergic, non-offensive, non-irritating, thus causing no harm to either partner's sex organs. if the male penis is thick and long but the vaginal cavity is too narrow to admit penetration or when there is extreme pain when penis is inserted into the vagina. The matter of fact is that during the course of pre-coitai play (or foreplay), the vaginal fluids lubricate the vagina canal profusely, when use of any sort of lubrication is hardly called for. Moreover, vagina is such a cosy, freshy, tender and muscular organ which has the capacity to enlarge itself to such an extent that length and thickness of penis is hardly of any consequence, as the vagina, due to its flexibility can admit any 'size of penis'. In one or two initial sexual unions, there may be some pain during insertion of penis but, due to its quality of adaptability, the vagina adjusts itself accordingly. When the penis penetration can be done without an difficulty, there is hardly any need to the use of any lubricant but, if the situation warrants, there is hardly any justification or need for avoiding use of any harmles, and agreeable lubricant.

Lights

Most males prefer to perform coitus in bright light, the reason being that female's body organs are visible and so that they can see, play, touch and kiss her sex arousing organs, and also watch their partner's reaction, intensity of enjoyment, her response etc. But, bright lights may be avoided, instead, light pink coloured lights be preferably used. Dark red, blue or violet lights should be avoided, unless there is a compelling preference for such colours. Women often prefer to have Coitus in the dark or else under very dim lights where only shade of physical forms are visible. Anyway, use of lights, colour and the duration of use, should necessarily be governed by personal likings and preferences. Some couples prefer 'Zero' power bulbs during the coital period.

Porno Movies

Some couples are used to watching porno movies to arouse passions. It gives them an instant turn on, helps to know novel postures of coitus. In most cases, some couples opt to perform entire sexual exercise, in accordance with scenes depicted in movie performed as per actions of the porno movie actors, tle vmsualising couples lose the sense of intensity and personal touch, as personal interaction and preferences get relegated to the hind seat. Porno movie viewing causes distraction of mind which takes away sensual pleasure. Further, some couples may reach orgasm too soon to enjoy the pleasures of ejaculation at the final climax. Some postures may be more practical on the screen and may cause physical harm to private parts of the couples. Premature ejaculation is often outcome which leaves most women on the verge of orgasm, but not complete orgasm. Men's purpose is served by viewing porno, movies but their female partners don't get a turn-on which factor causes an abrupt end to sex act, much to the disgust of the female partners.

Touch

Diane Ackerman says, "Feeling (of Touch) does not take place in the top most layer of the skin but in the second layer. This is why safe-crackers are sometimes shown sand-papering their finger prints." In any area of the body where there are more blood vessels and nerve endings, greater potential for stimulative sexuality is found. Erotic Zones pertain genitals, mouth, earlobes, breasts, inner thighs and buttocks. Not only such body parts but feet, stomach, palms and neck are also erotic spots. More men consider their women's thighs as an erogenous zone.

There is no denying the fact that sequence of touch is bound to have profound erotic effect. If less sensitive zones are touched first, and then gradually moving to the more sensitive erogenous

areas of the body, it will yield a brilliant turn-on. If, on the contrary, the most sensitive are worked upon first, it may (as it often does) result in turn off. Let the touch method be applied in the ascending order—that is to say to first touch the less sensitive areas and then moving to other more sensitive zones. We elaborate the said point. If food is churned, masticated slowly, saliva will mingle with it,

rendering its acceptable to the body. Similarly, if you go slow on touching methods, your juices and endocrine glands' secretions will help you getting complete taste (pleasure), and your body will get attuned to all the sensuality element generated by touch.

There are differences in the ways men and women prefer to be touched. Anna Moir and David jessel are of the view that "Women seem to be far more sensitive to pressure on skin, although they don't take longer than men to get aroused, as is widely believed. Many prefer a gentler touch at first, because of this greater sensitivity. But since people usually touch their lovers the way they like to be touched, you may need to show to your partner exactly how much pressure you want."

If you learn the art of timing into your mate's sexual senses and also those of your own, it is quite necessary for both of you not be a victim of habit. When any act is done in a routine manner our process of love-making is bound to be a drab monotony and even a turn-off. The most important part of love-making is that we all differ from each others' response and the person we wish to cohabitate with, can have varied sensations, reactions and enjoyments, from time-to-time, day-to-day.

Taste and Sensuality

We have about ten thousand taste buds that are grouped on our tongues by the kind of taste those are able to sense : Sour on the sides, bitter at back side and sweet at the tip, but the saltish taste can be perceived and sensed from (almost) any part of our tongue. When our skin is not properly cleaned, it also tastes mildly salty. So, tongue and skin have mild saltish taste. Moir and Jessel say, "Women are more sensitive to better flavours and also like higher concentrations of sweetness." Leaving aside preference for a particular type of taste, both men and women never prefer, rather despise, unpleasant tastes and foul odours. You don't have to use heavy deodorants and perfumes in bed as they are capable to cause instant turn-off. Only clean taste, in mouth and anywhere else in the body that can turn-on and prove erotic.

Seductive Sounds

Words express our feelings and emotions and lovers have great penchant for seductive sounds and adulatory words. When emotions run high and mouth fails to express feelings, eyes reveal the expressions. Sounds of pleasure, during sex, can also be erotic. Many people are inhibited about making noise in bed and as a result miss out on something that can enhance their pleasure and also their partners." If love notes are not reciprocated by the other partner (as) "I also love you," one is liable to get angry than turned-on. Let us admit that viable and congenial atmosphere do play great part in erotica. Any move that causes or aroused any sort of erotic feeling is, by far, the best sex arousal technique.

Erotic sounds and adulatory averments can be exchanged when mind is at peace, there is no disturbance, fear or obstacle. You can't enjoy sex under fear-psychosis. You can't even enjoy sex with tense egoistic and unpleasant approach. Be happy, remain happy, and also look happy—no amount of remorse should evern find a way into your bed-room. The more carefree you are, the more relaxed you stay.

HOW TO ENHANCE MALE SEX DESIRE

It is not always possible to enjoy coital climax—the reasons vary from person to person. An astute operator keeps his technical know-how fully updated. He equally cares for upkeep of the apparatus he is handling. Instead of passing on the blame to any other person (in sex context, say your wife or a woman), first weigh your own self, have a full self-appraisal and after finding out the lacuna, try to mend the fault.

You should be more conscious of what your partner is averse to, hates, dislikes or abhors. She has her own problems, perhaps, and when such problems compound, both should sit together and discuss every minute point. Let there be no element, not even an inkling of taking the other partner's views as amiss. Try to understand and appreciate the problems of your female partner.

The husband (or any male for that matter) should keep the following guidelines in view:

- ☞ Remain tension free. Never attempt any coitus when the mind is disturbed. You will do well to disclose your problem to your wife, take her into confidence and seek her advice.
- ☞ Intercourse should always be done in an airy, neat,

clean, fully ventilated room, free from any encroachment and disturbance. If both partners agree, let there be a zero watt red bulb whose red light will flare up passions and impart added enjoyment to your sex fervour.

- ☞ Ensure personal hygiene. Use deodorants, scents to ward off foul smelling body odours.
- ☞ Before sex, have a bath or at least, sponge your whole body, particularly your ears, nose, arm pits, inner thighs, prepuce and glans penis. Spray some pleasing scent on whole body to enjoy an added erotic feeling.
- ☞ Give equal opportunity to your partner to have her own time. Never hurry her. Any act done in a hurry will take away charm of sex.
- ☞ Never plunge yourself at once into intercourse. Foreplay should be an essential forerunner to any sex act. Foreplay is a reliable method to prepare your partner for the coming event. Let her also have her own way. Never act like a dictator or a super human.
- ☞ Persuade your partner. Appreciate and endear each and every organ of her body, even if you don't have fancy to some of her organs. Tell her that she is not, in any way, inferior to Aishwarya or any film actress. Such loving compliments and endearments would help her to active participation.
- ☞ Aggression, rough-shod treatment, demeaning, slighting or insulting will have a rebound reaction, resulting an imposed coitus.
- ☞ Excite her gently, carefully, slowly, tenderly. If she resists and forbids you not to touch any one or more of her sex organs, abide by her wishes and never force your way to compel her to mental withdrawal and physical inertia.
- ☞ If, for any reason whatsoever, she is disinclined for sex act, you can lie down together and discuss some subject of common interest. The chances are that during course of interaction, she may get ready and

herself invite you for sex act.

- ☞ Try to avoid sex during advance stage of pregnancy, during menstruation or when she is having leucorrhoea. But sex act must be given a good-bye, if either of the partners is suffering from AIDS, HIV any venereal infection, asthmatic bout (attack), high fever, any infectious/contagious disease.
- ☞ Fondle, caress, cuddle, kiss, pamper each and every erogenous zone—but very slowly. During the course of foreplay she, herself, would guide you, as to on which sex organs she wishes, rather prefers, to be touched.
- ☞ Give equal chance to your partner to indulge in sex act. She should play inactive role in the whole play, and successful intercourse ensues from joint efforts of both partners.
- ☞ If you are about to reach the climax, you should let your partner know a bit earlier so that she could help you to delay orgasm, by adopting 'squeeze the tempo' method Moreover, she will also get mentally prepared to face the problem of your early ejaculation.
- ☞ After you have reached your climaxed orgasm, you should never leave her in-between. Wait till she also reaches her orgasm. You should not ever prove to be a selfish sex performer, as her sentiments deserve to be respected.

Above mentioned points deserve to be modified as per mutual consent and convenience. Indian women are shy and reserve, they rarely give vent to their feelings, and this is more true of those women who are confined within confines of four walls of their house. So, both the partners should try to respect each other's likes and dislikes, desires and aversions, physical compulsion and constraints, to enjoy real bliss of sexual intercourse.

Organs and Foreplay

An orgasm represents the zenith of human pleasurable experiences. Orgasm is derived from the Greek word orgies, which means to swell with lust.

Orgasm is defined as an explosive, cerebrally encoded, neuromuscular response, at the peak of sexual arousal by psychopathological stimuli, the pleasurable sensations of which are experienced in association with dispensable pelvic physiological concomitants.

Why orgasm?

Sex is not merely the means to an end. It is both: the means to an end (procreation), as well as and end in itself (pleasure). Orgasm is nature's masterstroke. By providing an inherently sensual pleasure-oriented side to our personality, nature has ingeniously accomplished the dual objective of pleasure and procreation.

The pleasure principle has, is, and shall always, remain principal.

Early Orgasmic Response (EOR)

This is defined as an orgasm that is experienced earlier than one's idealized expectations, which are within rational limits.

Delayed Orgasmic Response (DOR)

When orgasm does ultimately occur, but is delayed beyond one's idealized expectations, which are within rational limits, it is called delayed orgasmic response.

Impaired Orgasmic Response (IOR)

It is defined as a reduction in the intensity of the orgasmic pleasure.

Absent Orgasmic Response (AOR)

This category includes cases in which there is complete failure to experience pleasure.

How does one reach orgasm?

When an individual has a sexual desire he departs from the normal state and enters into the sexual state and is deemed to have undergone sexual grounding. Sexual grounding or the sexual state is a state in which the subject becomes receptive to the perception of stimuli inputs as sexual. Once this occurs, psychopathological stimuli arouse the sex center in the brain which starts sending out impulses, which are usually pleasurable. When such impulses reach the genitalia, the resultant increased flow of blood leads to congestion in genitals. This phenomenon is usually manifested as erection in the male and lubrication in the female. Further stimulation enhances arousal and eventually culminates in orgasm.

What is interplay?

Interplay encompasses the whole spectrum of sexual interaction, that is, the entire grommet of motions and emotions between individuals indulging in "play".

Is foreplay important?

Yes, it is extremely important. It kindles the desire and marks the beginning of the interplay. Adequate foreplay ensures adequate arousal and promotes sexual compatibility.

Is afterplay important?

Yes. Afterplay is as important as foreplay. Though penovaginal sex is regarded as the most intimate and satisfying form of sexual activity, this is not always true. There are many women who report "I am not worried about orgasm but I would very much appreciate a bit of love play. Vatsyayan, in the Kamasutra, has given a lot of emphasis to afterplay and he has mentioned that afterplay is equally, if nor more, important than foreplay. Most people enjoy being held, cuddled, talked to, and partners need to communicate with each other as to what they prefer. Many a time, a woman in her fifties or so would come and report: "Doctor, sex is now far more satisfying despite the fact that my husband is unable to achieve erection." Perhaps he forced to learn or devote more time to foreplay and afterplay which takes away the feeling of mechanical sex and, at times, when he is unable to perform, there is enough warmth and affection.

Foreplay introduces and afterplay summarizes the crucial interplay.

Some others call it PARAM SUKH (Eternal Happiness).

Are there any techniques to delay orgasm?

Many techniques have been used to delay orgasm. The methods commonly used by many include mental arithmetic, local anaesthetic ointment, wearing a disposable tissue and a condom around the penis to decrease sensitivity.

Other methods include:

1. Voluntarily interrupting and restarting the flow of urine repeatedly.
2. Vajroli mudra and Ashwini mudra.
3. The squeezes / stop-start technique.

How does one go ahead with these exercises?

Identifying the pelvic muscles is simple. Just voluntarily interrupt and restart the flow of urine. These are the muscles you need to train. Once identified, try contracting and relaxing these muscles five times, thrice a day; increase the frequency to ten times in the next week and then, 15 and 20 times in subsequent weeks. Continue repetitions thrice a day 20 times for four to six weeks. These exercises can be done whilst standing at the bus stop, sitting in the office or at any other time. After contracting the pelvic muscles, one should hold them for about 3 seconds before relaxation's and 60 or 70 of these exercise maneuvers in a day can lead to benefits in six to eight weeks' time.

Are there any exercises for enhancing the male sexual performance?

Exercises to strengthen the pelvic muscles (chiefly those surrounding the penis) help to achieve better control over the orgasmic reflex, improve the quality or orgasm and also increase the circulation of blood in the pelvic area, perhaps leading to better erectly ability.

Which yogic exercise helps delay the climax?

The Vajroli mudra and the Ashwini mudra could be of help in the treatment of early orgasmic response. In Vajroli mudra, a person sits in any comfortable meditative asana, places his hands on his knees, closes his eyes, relaxes and breathes through his nose. After a deep inhalation, he holds his breath and tries to draw the sexual organs upward by pulling and tensing the lower abdomen and contracting the pelvic muscles. These contractions are similar to those when one has an urge to pass urine but wishes to hold on for some time. In Ashwini mudra, a person sits in the Padmasana (lotus position) or any meditative pose, relaxes the whole body, closes the eyes, inhale deeply, hold the breath, bends the head forward and presses the chin tightly against the chest (chin-lock position). He then contracts the anal sphincter and relaxes, and repeats this procedure a few times. Then he extends the neck (unlocks the chin), exhales and simultaneously relaxes the sphincter. These yogic exercises strengthen the anterior and posterior parts of the pubo-coccygeul muscles, respectively. Such exercises, when done ten times, every morning and evening, for six to eight weeks often lead to adequate control over the orgasmic reflex. Sometimes, the practice of contracting the anterior part of the pubo-coccygeul muscle just prior to orgasmic (ejaculatory) inevitability during coitus helps delay the orgasm (climax).

Orgasm and Roller

If arousal takes place without release it is likely to cause discomfort. That discomfort can best be handled through mutual expression of care and affirmation.

If you are a woman who consistently experiences arousal without release it is crucial that you share this with your husband. Let him know what your body feels like so that the two of you can move closer together. There can be some relief even in being reached out to. He needs to know what you need.

What about multiple orgasms?

A woman's body is designed so that she can have another orgasm at any point of the resolution phase. It can be five seconds, five minutes or fifty minutes after the previous orgasm. There is no waiting or rest period necessary before she is physically capable of experiencing another orgasm if the stimulation is continued or renewed. Her body does not need to return to its prestimulated state before it can be responsive again. This is not to say that having more than one orgasm is better or those sexually "together" women will desire this. The point is that, physically, if she desires it and can allow it; the woman's orgasm can be repeated indefinitely.

For the Man

After orgasmic release, the man returns rather quickly to the prestimulated state. His erection may not decrease completely, but the penis is usually somewhat flaccid and the testicles lower. There is a loss in the tension build-up and in the intensity of the feelings. Some men report that the glans or head of the penis becomes very sensitive to touch after an ejaculation and that because of this they want to quickly disengage from their partner. The man may not have told this to his wife because he feels uncomfortable or embarrassed about it. It is important to know that a significant number of men feel this post ejaculation pain. If you experience this discomfort, it is crucial to share this with your partner so that she be sympathetic and understanding, rather than taking your withdrawal as a kind of rejection.

It is rare for a man not to experience orgasm. However, there are some men (especially older men) who do not need an orgasm and who do not feel frustrated without one.

Different Disorders and Sexual Life

In our life, we all suffer from different diseases, time to time. All these common disorders does not affect the sex life but diseases like diabetes affect it. Findout more information:

What are the most common sexual dysfunctions among diabetics?

Erectile dysfunctions are common amongst diabetics. The causes could be vascular, neurological or psychological. In diabetic impotence, the history is suggestive of the presence of desire but decline in erectile ability at all times. Usually, the onset is gradual. In some, the presenting symptom could be premature ejaculation and rarely retrograde ejaculation. Diabetic women sometimes complain of reduction in lubrication and difficulty in reaching orgasm. Monilial infection may further reduce lubrication and associated itching makes intercourse uncomfortable. Monilial infection often leads to balanitis (inflammation of the glans penis).

What limits should one observe?

There is nothing like a limit in sex, either you indulge or you do not. A heart attack could have occurred even otherwise, like while passing urine or going to the toilet. However, the best person to advise you would be a cardiologist because the treatment needs to be tailored according to individual needs. The following precautions may be useful—

(1) Avoid clandestine sexual activity as it tends to increase the heart rate more than usual.
(2) Avoid elaborate meals and alcohol prior to the sex act as lot of energy and blood flow would be utilized for digestion.
(3) It is advisable to do regular physical exercise, so that sexual exercise need not be an unaccustomed exertion.
(4) One may keep a nitroglycerine tablet or spray handy, if anticipating chest pain.

Is the female superior position advantageous to males with cardiac problems?

Scientific research has proved that alternation in sexual positions such as taking the bottom position or assuming a passive role has no significant energy saving advantage. The blood pressure and heart rates have been directly measured and have been found to be almost the same in men in the male superior as well as the female superior positions. The same holds true for females with cardiac problems.

Has high blood pleasure anything to do with sex ?

There is a marked increase in blood pressure during sexual intercourse. Very high blood pressure does pose a danger of cerebral haemorrhage and mycordial infection. However, it is desirable to control high blood pressure. Once controlled, the danger of catastrophic event is negligible with the short-terms changes that occur during intercourse and other physical activities. It is equally, if not more, important to inform the patients about the likely side-effects of anti-hypertensive drugs on their sexual response.

Which anti-hypertensive medicines have the least sexual side effects ?

No generalization can be made. However, diuretics, ACE inhibitors and vacillators have the least sexual side-effects. Yoga and Transcendental Meditation with biofeed back could be a safe adjunct.

"Whatever anti-hypertensive medications I use, my sex desire and potency get reduces... What should I do.... reduce

the dose, stop the drug or stop sex ?"

Consult a competent physician. On most occasions, the medication can be changed to a drug which has the same effect on the target symptom, without polarizing the sexual system.

What precautions should one take during coitus if one is suffering from bronchial asthma?

The sex act per se is not very stressful. Shortness of breath is a natural response during the sex act and more so if one suffers from bronchial asthma. It becomes more intense if accompanied by anxiety. Use of a bronchodilator prior to sexual activity could be helpful.

What sexual problems can a man with kidney failure have ?

He may have less desire and inadequate erection due to anaemia, uraemia and testicular dysfunction. Like in any other chronic disease, psychological problems like depression and anxiety, leading to decline in sexual desire, are common.

What is Peyronie's disease ?

This is an uncommon condition usually found in men who are in their fifties and above. A fibrous plaque develop in the penis, leading to curvature of the penis which become apparent during erection. It may cause discomfort and, at times, pain during intercourse. Usually, this is a self-limiting disease. Operative procedures are rarely resorted to.

What are the causes of blood in semen ?

Any condition which can give rise to congestion and inflammation of the prostate and seminal vesicles can lead to blood in semen. Trauma and urethritis may also lead to blood in semen.

Can hepatitis (jaundice) lead to sexual problems ?

Yes, it kills the appetite for sex. In addition, the fear of transmitting or acquiring the disease (Type B) via sexual contact adds anxiety to the existing problem.

Can one indulge in sex during jaundice ?

This will depend upon the cause of jaundice. Of the many causes of jaundice, the one that should cause maximum concern is viral hepatitis, the reason being the sexual transmission of the disease to the spouse, who then may or may not manifest jaundice but may yet harbour the virus. Roughly speaking, the changes of transmitting the virus are maximum in the early stages of illness, especially in the programme phase which immediately precedes the onset of jaundice. The Hepatitis 'B' virus and possibly 'C' and 'D' virus being the important culprits, it would be prudent to consult the physician at the earliest and get both the partners investigated for the same.

Vaginal and even oral sex may transmit the virus. Barrier contraception (condom) does provide an effective method of protection against the sexual transmission; however, it would still be advisable to get the spouse vaccinated at the earliest as per the expert's advice.

Once the patient with jaundice has developed immunity (antibodies) to the virus and the spouse is already protected (with vaccination which takes up to weeks), normal sexual intercourse can be resumed.

Hepatitis D (delta) does not require any additional vaccination apart from that for Hepatitis B. Hepatitis C is rarely transmitted due to sexual contact. Using barrier contraception during sexual activity is advisable.

How does arthritis affect sexual relationships ?

In arthritis, pain and deformity usually lead to difficulty in the sex act, especially when the hip, knees or the back are involved. Factors like frustration, anger, dependency and low self-image due to deformity lead to depression. Steroid side-effects, e.g., obesity and moon-face complement this depression. Thus, arthritis debilitates sexual relationships both physically as well mentally.

What are the treatment options available ?

Discussion with the partner about alternatives and more comfortable positions is the best option. Speak to your partner about the areas which arouse you the most and inform him / her about the painful areas. Plan your drug schedule in such a way that you take pain relievers prior to the sex act. Select the best time for coitus, i.e., osteoarthritis is at its worst in the evening and better in the morning and the reverse is true for rheumatoid arthritis. This precaution will make the sexual encounter more comfortable. A shower or a tub bath together with warm water will act as a good foreplay activity, in additional to diminishing stiffness and pain. Use of lubricants can enhance the pleasure. It is particularly useful in Sjogren's syndrome, where along with a reduction of other secretion of the body, there is a reduction in vaginal lubrication. Advice will vary with individual cases.

Can a man have sexual intercourse after a prostate operation ?

Yes, he can. Currently, the greatest number of prostatectomies are done via the transurethra route. After surgery, the quality of erection remains the same at the time of climax and men experience the same pleasure. The ejaculation usually remains unaffected though, in some individual, the quantity of ejaculate outside may be less or absent because of retrograde ejaculation.

What is the effect of mastectomy on a woman's sexuality ?

Though anatomically mutilating, theoretically a radical masterdom should have no effect on a woman's sexuality as her physiology remain unchanged. However, the physical mutilation may wreak a psychological trauma which can affect a woman's self-image and self-esteem to a great extent. She may begin to harbour the feeling that she has become less feminine and hence less attractive. This feeling may depress her and make her withdraw from social and sexual contacts. The surgeon must explain to the patient the operative procedure, the interpretive risks, the possible outcome and that it is being performed as a potentially life-saving curative / palliative procedure. To patients who are very apprehensive about the disfigurement, the surgeon may explain that reconstructive mammoplasty can be performed if so desired.

Can a woman lead a normal sex life after hysterectomy ?

Yes. Women who are sexually active before hysterectomy continue to remain so even after the surgery. Sexual life remains unchanged, as the coital function is preserved. Hysterectomy usually involves the removal of the uterus, but if it necessitates the removal of the ovaries as well, then the patient may require hormone supplementation.

Is there any relation between sex and obesity ?

On the face of it, sex and obesity may have no connection at all. Often sexual inadequacy may lead to anxiety and/ or depression which may result in increased food intake in some individual. Hormonal disturbances may also lead to obesity. This factory may produce interference with normal sexual functioning and lead to overall sluggish behaves. Sedentary habits and lack of exercise are common in obese individuals. This lifestyle may result in flabby muscles and sexual pleasure may decrease when the specific muscles that play a part in love making get easily fatigued.

Can smoking hinder sexually response ?

Smoking results in construction of the blood vessels, leading to an inadequate supply of blood to the genital organs which may, in turn, lead to sexual inadequacy. Discontinuation of smoking by a heavy smoker leads to an increase in the desire and many have reported better erectile ability.

Do routine X-rays induce impotence ?

No

Are there any diseases associated with increased sexual desire ?

Increase in sexual desire can be seen during mania where there is acceleration of activity in all spheres. Sometimes, there is increased sexual desire in schizophrenic patients, perhaps because of loss of inhibitors. Organic diseases, like a tumour in the frontal lobe of the brain or disturbances following head injuries or the post-octal stage following an epileptic attack, may be associated with increased sexual desire.

Is masturbation after marriage normal ?

Yes. Masturbation is normal even in married individual. It may be encouraged during period of separation, illness and in conditions where one partner's sexual needs are beyond the sexual capacity of the other.

What physical changes occur in the sexual apparatus when one grows older ?

As a man grows older, erection takes a longer time to occur. Similarly, in women, lubrication takes a longer time to occur. A man may often required direct physical stimulation to achieve erection and the same task also true of a woman's lubrication. With the passage of time, the colour of the semen changes from white to light yellow, the consistency gets thinner and the quantity decreases. When people are not informed about these facts, anxiety can be generated, as there is a vast discrepancy between the unrealistic expectation and the real experience. This factor hampers the sexual response, leading to avoidance of sexual overtures. Older persons tend to become obese because of sedentary lives, lack of exercise and changes in hormonal levels. Exercises to tone up the muscles and good functioning to beautify are essential. Such exercises help in improving the self-image and promotion of a better sex life.

What are the most common conditions which could decrease one's sex drive in the later years ?

The common reasons for a reduced sex drive in later years are :

- Monotony and lack of interest
- Changes in physical appearance.
- Misconception about one's warning sexuality.
- Lack of communication.
- Depression.

Does the female sexual desire increase or decrease at menopause ?

Some women report an increase, while others report a decrease, in sexual desire at menopause. Increase in sexual desire may be because of relative freedom from pregnancy and, hence, one may reopens and perform with greater enthusiasm. Some women harbour the misconception that menopause marks the end of their sexual career and this fear increases their sexual drives as an affirmation of their femininity. Menopause (or even a few years earlier), a reduction in the secretion of the ovarian hormones may cause atrophy of the vaginal epithelium which leads to reduction in lubrication and hence pain at the time of sexual intercourse. This development causes a decline in sexual desire and a woman tends to avoid sexual overtures.

Is oestrogen therapy at menopause safe ?

It is advisable to consult a gynaecologist for the use of hormornal preposition during menopause. Oestraogen replacement can avoid atrophic vaginites which leads to painful intercourse and can also help in preventing osteoporosis which usually leads to frequent fractures. It would be best to take oestrogen with progesterone in monthly cycles.

Does benign prosthetic hyperbolas (BPH) increase libido ?

No. it does not increase libido.

Which sexual position is useful to individual with localized low back pain ?

The affected partner should lie on his / her back with the hips flexed. In this posture, the muscles are relaxed and the vertebral column remains flat on the bed; hence this position is comfortable.

Can obese individuals be helped in matters of sexual activity ?

Extreme obesity primarily inhibits sexual pleasure on account of mechanical inreference. Side-by-side positions where neither partner bears the other's weight and, at the same time, has all limbs free from embrance, can be advantageously.

Which positions are comfortable for the woman during late pregnancy ?

The lateral positions are generally found to be more comfortable.

Doctor, is there any sexual position which allows better grip ?

Yes, the rear entry (doggie) position and the woman's

legs crossed position allow better grip as compared to other solutions. In the woman's legs crossed position, the intercourse is performed in the missionary position, where later, the woman crosses and keeps her legs inside her male partner's legs. This enhances arousal and both these positions are helpful in those males who face difficulty in reaching orgasm.

What is meant by retarded ejaculation ? Does diabetes have a part to play in cases of retarded ejaculation ?

Retarded ejaculation is the opposite of premature ejaculation. Western researchers observed that undetected diabetes is the most common cause of impotence. Diabetes may also cause ejaculatory disturbance, but it seems to impair the erectile mechanism more poundal, or at least equal.

This history is absolutely essential and, in a large number of individuals suffering from sexual inadequacy, ignorance about the sex act may be a major factor. Adequate explanation about the act of coitus and methods to enhance orgasmic pleasure may improve the majority cases.

What could be the reason for buckling of penis during penetetration ?

Such buckling usually takes places because of reduced axial pressure following trauma or fracture of penis. In this condition all tests, including NPTR and Doppler will be normal but the patient will give a history of bending / buckling of penis at any attempt .

Are people with a single testicle impotent ?

No. A single "normal" testicle secretes enough hormones to maintain an individual's vitality.

What is the most common cause of erectile dysfunction ?

An occasional episode of an erectile failure, due to functional or situations like fatigue, tension or pressure to respond bad perform, is one of the common causes of erectile disfunction. This anxiety, fire-lived during subsequent, similar encounter, would result in related failures.

How can one distinguish a psychological erectile problem from an organic one?

If a man reports an erection of adeuqte quality and sustenance in one situation and not in another, one can conclude that the problem is largely psychological.

Can alcohol lead to impotence ?

Yes.

How does one treat alcohol-induced impotence?

The treatment programme needs to be tailored according to individual needs and circumstances. The physician must determine whether the sexual dysfunction is connected with an isolated episode of drinking or is related to the long-term consumption of alcohol. He must confirm the status of the erectile and ejaculator components after history taking and a careful physical examination. If the impotence is secondary to an isolated episode of alcohol intake, then the physician may reassure the patient that the sexual function may revert to normal if the latter completely abstains from alcohol. He should also then be made aware that his preoccupation with fear of failure can hamper his sexual responses. Necessary sexual techniques, with adequate blending of supportive psychotherapy and behaviour modification, may prove extremely beneficial. It is advisable to counsel the partner as well. She could be of great help in the treatment programme if she can understand the situation and is prepared to provide the supportive atmosphere.

What are the most common causes of organic impotence ?

Diabetes, vascular disorders and radical cancer surgeries of the abdomen and pelvis are amongst the most common causes of organic impotence.

Is semen analysis necessary in a patient affected by impotence ?

Absolutely not. The absence or deficiency of sperms neither indicates nor results in impotence. Sterility and virility are two entirely different concepts and depend upon different types of cells present in the tests.

Which investigations are helpful in the diagnosis of sexual dysfunctions ?

Along with metabolic, hormonal and routine physical examination, one should also check the tone of the anal sphincter. Evaluation of the autonomic nervous system is a must in cases of impotence. The following procedures are important -

NPT monitoring : Nocturnal penile tumescence monitoring can help in determining whether one is getting erections or not. This procedure, however, does not give any idea about the rigidity of the penis.

NPTR monitoring : This procedures along with the preceding one gives an idea also about rigidity and sustenance of the erection.

EMG : Electromyographic studies could help diagnose neurological lesions causing impotence and reduction in pleasure and squirting of semen at the time of orgasm.

Intrapenile injection : This procedure involves an injection of vasoactive drugs (Papaverine, Papaverine mixed with Chlorpromazien or Phenotolamin, Prostag land in E_1) directly into the lateral aspect of the penis. Depending upon the erectile response which the patent has and the amount of drugs which is injected gives a conceal a clue to diagnose inorganic, psychogenic or vasculogenic erectile dysfunction.

Doppler examination : This is a non-invasive technique which helps in determining the potency of the superficial and deep blood vessels of the penis. Its graphic representation are useful in judging the blood flow. On colour Doppler, blood flow can be clearly visualized.

Penile blood pressure : Penile systole blood pressure (by using a Doppler probe and a special cuff tied round the penis) divided by the systolic blood pressure of the arm, gives the penile bronchial index (PBI). If the reading is abnormal, it is probably indicative of vascular insufficiency.

Infusion cavernosometry and cavernosography

Infusion studies with normal saline are helpful in diagnosing venous leaks responsible for inadequate erection. Cavernosography with a contrast medium helps in detecting the presence of abnormal drainage channels responsible for erectile inadequacy.

What is an Aphrodisiac (Sex Tonic)

"Aphrodisiacs" are foods, herbs, potions, or drugs which are believed to increase sexual desire and improve sexual performance. Aphrodisiacs are named after the Greek goddess of love Aphrodite. The belief is sex tonics to stimulate one's sexuality is as old as the human race. Different aphrodisiacs have been in vogue at different times. In the 1960s, an Oriental herb called ginseng was very popular. The root of this plant became the largest selling aphrodisiac in the American market. In the 1970s, "royal jelly" became a popular energizer for the gonads. Later on, vitamin E and zinc became the most commonly accepted nutritional aphrodisiacs.

How do aphrodisiacs work?

Sex tonics usually "work" in three ways. Some like alcohol and marijuana, alter the mental state; others increase the flow of blood to the genital apparatus, e.g., yohimbine and some others cause severe irritation and inflammation of the genitourinary tract, e.g., Spanish fly. Sex tonics, as such, have no effect on sexuality. The most effective mode of action is the well-known mechanism of suggestion. The fact remains that no food or drug on earth has as yet been to be a direct sex stimulant.

What is the effect of alcohol on sexual functioning?

Alcohol is essentially a central nervous system

depressant. In small doses, it gives a feeling of warmth and well-being and removes social inhibitions which probably accounts for its popularity as an aphrodisiac. However, as mentioned, "The desire it provokes, but takes away the performance" is unfortunately yet undisputed true.

What are the long-term effects of alcohol on an individual's sexual functioning?

Chronic alcoholism impairs the sexual functioning due to many causes. The repeated impairment of response and performance during acute episodes of alcohol intake create anxiety which proves to be a "psychological barrier" to responses and performance in subsequent sexual encounters also.

Besides, chronic alcoholism results in hepatic and neurological damage. This damage leads to decreased sensitivity and impotence in the male and early menopause, excessive menstrual and intermenstrual bleeding in the female and an overall decrease in sexual desire in both sexes.

Is marijuana a sexual stimulant?

Though it has been experimented extensively all over the world, the use of marijuana as an aphrodisiac is unpredictable and the effects are largely because of reduction of inhibition, increased suggestibility and a time distortion effect.

What are the sexual effects of cocaine?

Cocaine leads to a temporary increase in sexual excitability but along with this feeling, it also leads to flight of ideas, fear reaction and paranoid thinking.

What is testosterone?

Testosterone is a natural androgen produced by the Leydig cells of the testes in men. If the cells do not function, puberty is delayed and sexual infantilism persists. If these cells fail later in life, i.e., after puberty, a man experiences loss of libido and potency, a reduced ejaculate, a gradual decrease in testicular size and slow growing facial hair.

What is your opinion about testosterone in the treatment of sexual dysfunctions?

Testosterone is often used for its "supposed" aphrodisiac effect. However, it is seldom effective and is useful only in those exceptional cases where there is a genuine lack of testosterone in the body or where there is evidence of failure in the development of secondary sexual characteristics or during old age when there is evidence of low levels of testosterone. If used irrationally in young individuals, it may cause a decrease in the sperm count. Abnormal liver functions and cases of liver malignancy have also been reported. If administered in females, hirsutism, the male pattern of baldness, enlargement of the clitoris and deepening of the voice are the chief side-effects. Abnormalities of the glucose tolerance curve (the test for diabetes) may be encountered and disurbances could occur in previously stable diabetes. Testosterone is often used, empirically, to improve sexual desire and performance in middle-aged men. However, a significant decrease in testosterone secretion in middle-aged men is very uncommon.

While using testosterone for the elderly, it is advisable to do a rectal examination prior to its use, as testosterone can precipitate malignancy of the prostate gland. Unless the symptoms reveal, and metabolic investigations confirm a deficiency of testosterone, it should never be used.

What is papaverine?

Papaverine is a drug that acts as a vasodilator and muscle relaxant. Direct injection of the drug into the penis will result in a firm and relatively long-lasting erection.

Which are the other drugs used in the injection erection therapy?

Phantomlike, chlorpromazine and prostate land in E, can be used in combination with papaverine. Prostate land in E, can also be used alone.

Are there any side-effects of using papaverine?

Sometimes the erection achieved by the papaverine injection fails to subside. Hence, this drug should be used with caution. One should avoid using papaverine more than twice a week, as it may lead to scarring, bruising, etc. Long-term use may cause fibrosis and curvature of the penis. The drug also suffers from the disadvantage of losing its effect over a period of time. It should be used only under a physician's guidance.

What are the modern medicines commonly used that can paralyse the sexual system?

Modern medicine, if indiscriminately used, can play havoc with the sexual system. Over-the-counter medicines, easy accessibility and self-medication have made many a drug liable for potential abuse. In my experience, the drugs commonly used that could be detrimental in terms of sexual health are the following-

- Antihypertensives: Reserpine (rawolfia alkaloid), beta-blockers, alpha-methyl dopa, ganglion-blocking agents.
- Antiandrogens: Cimetidine, ketoconazole, spironolactone.
- Anticonvulsants: Barbiturates, carbamazepine.
- Anticholinergics: Belladonna alkaloids.
- Antipsychotics, Antidepressants, and antianxiety group of drugs.

In such cases, the medication can be changed to drugs which have the same effect on the target symptom without paralysing the sexual system.

What is Viagra?

Vigara, pharmacologically known as sildenafil Citrate, is an oral drug preparation for the treatment of the erectile dysfunction. It is used for the treatment of men who have difficulty in maintaining an erection.

Is it a true aphrodisiac?

Yes and no. In other words, it does not create an erection but can enhance an already achieved erection.

How is it available?

It is available in 25 mg, 50 mg and 100 mg potency, only on the production of a prescription and not over the counter.

What is the mechanism of action?

For understanding the mechanism of action, it is essential to know the physiology of penile erection, which involves the release of a chemical mediator that increases the blood flow to the penis, resulting in an erection. Viagara enhances the effect of this chemical mediator, thereby enhancing the erection. Thus, it enhanes an already achieved erection and does not create an erection.

What are personal massagers? Are they useful?

"Personal massagers" are also known as vibrators. These vibrators can help in providing additional stimulation in some individuals. Some women prefer to hold a vibrator on the clitoris even during coitus. Most men prefer to use a vibrator with slow speed on the area around the scrotum and the underside of the penis. It is particularly helpful for older men as they require more intense physical stimulation as compared to younger men, and a vibrator could serve as a good adjunct.

Which is the best vibrator?

There are several models available, like the battery-operated ones and the electricity-operated ones with multiple attachments. However, one must not forget that at times even a finger could prove to be the best vibrator!

What is the best natural aphrodisiac?

The best natural aphrodisiac is an attractive and affectionate partner passionately asking to be enjoyed. The ideal aphrodisiac still eludes us, but the quest for it continues, as hope springs eternal.

What is the role of Ayurvedic medicines ?

Ayurvedic mediciens are best aphrodiacs with no side effects. The mixtures and powder prepared by well qualified physician are helpful in using most sex problems including impotency and premature ejaculation.

What advice would you give for leading a better sex life?

Sexual literacy is the primary requirement for a good sex life. Do not be under pressure to perform or respond. Try to get familiar with you own and your partner's anatomy. Communicate mutual likes and dislikes. Adequate communication is vital for a healthy and mutually satisfying sex life. Avoid being monotonous. Be innovative and try different positions. Devote adequate time for foreplay and after play. Remember sensual is sexual.

Avoid stress, smoking and alcohol. Proper weight, balanced diet, regular exercise and yoga are essential for a better sex life. What is good for the whole body is good for sex.

How do I Know When I Am Ready for a Relationship ?

Ask Yourself: Why would this person want to be with you? How considerate, independent, funny and interesting are you? Relationships of all kinds are the classrooms in which we learn all about life. "What makes live relationships so taxing is that there's the possibility to be hooked at the deepest level," say experts. Women often look to a man to complete them, particularly financially. But, the truth is that you need to have a deep relationship with yourself. Then, you can have one with others.

Be aware of self: Self-awareness includes recognising what pushes your buttons, and how you react in certain situations. It's important to learn to be a wife, a lover, a sister or a friend from your family of origin. The perceptions we have of these roles and the ways we reach out are programmed from birth. So, recalling your family's style of communication will give you an insight into your own way of operating.

Get over past realationships: This is crucial before embarking on a new relationship. Question where you are emotionally with regard to your previous relationships? If you don't do this, it doesn't matter who you choose, you will simply project everything you associate with the last man, on to the new one.

Take Responsibility for you choices: At the end of a relationship, you will go through a predictable sequence of emotions: denial, anger and then blame, which is where a lot of people get stuck. As long as you hold someone else accountable, you can't let go of the relationship. You need to take responsibility for your choices and stop pointing fingers. You may move into a state of depression where you mourn the loss of the connection, but when you realise that the relationship has been an opportunity to learn, you finally reach acceptance.

Learn from the past: Relationships of all kinds are the classrooms in which we need to learn from past mistakes and take care not to repeat them. That is when you are ready to move on.

Signs to know if your boyfriend loves you as much as you love him

- Focus on how you feel when you are loving. Does loving someone feel good regardless if it's returned? Is your loving someone conditional on them loving you back? If so, why?
- Do you feel loved when you partner isn't around? If not, why not? Do you accept yourself and appreciate your qualities?
- Are you doing things for your lover that you really don't want to do, but feel you need to, to keep their love? Are you doing things for them, expecting something in return? What are you expecting? And have you told them what that is?
- Have you talked to your partner about what things cause you to feel loved? Don't get caught up in "if they loved me, they'd know", because they don't think about these issues, and if he answers are no, you know it is one-sided.

How to ask your friend out for a date and not spoil your friendship?

- First, the best person to start to get romantically involved with, is someone that you are already good friends with. That is, a great friendship is really necessary for a great relationship. You should really enjoy each other's company, spending time together and doing things together. That's the whole reason you're a, couple, right? So, start with that whole mentality. This person is someone you want to be friends with and to get to know better.
- Start out like you would with any other friend. Learn about the things they like. If she loves horses, get a book on horses and learn about them too. Ask her questions about them. People who love a topic love to talk about the topic. If she adores Pintos she probably could talk to you about them for hours and hours. If he loves Mustangs, read up on Mustangs and ask him about the differences between the 1960s and the 1970s. You'll learn something in the process, and the more time, you spend together, the better your relationship!
- People always ask "What do we talk about". There's no magic formula - talk about snowflakes or talk about the weather. Best friends talk about things that they are interested in. Find out what this person's interests are, and talk about them!
- Once you're on speaking terms, and are comfortable talking to each other, then the next step of talking about going to see a movie that you're both interested in is pretty natural. You both take Spanish and like Spanish? You suggest that the two of you go see a Spanish movie when it comes around. It's far less stressful when it's a common interest, and you're both already used to talking about the topic.
- Now that you're doing things together. Step the emotional side up a notch. Friends hug each other hello and goodbye. So you're already doing that, right?

If not, start it up. If you are, then now give that hug with a soft kiss on the cheek. When You're walking, loan her your jacket or ask him to borrow his. The more you do these small things, the more normal it will be, and soon enough, the dates will be of the boyfriend-girlfriend variety.

Take it in stages, and it all works out easily!

Forbidden Love

A break from the tradition, not just in India but everywhere men dating older women is real, though rare. Ashton Kuchner's relationship with Hollywood diva Demi Moore has fetched him instant fame. The guy is so besotted with his ladylove that the age difference just doesn't matter. Among the Indian examples, we have the happy couple of Sachin and Anjali Tendulkar. But on the flip side, is the couple of Saif Ali Khan and Amrita who broke off recently. Whatever be the consequences, the inevitable happens when it does. Though it may sound against the tide and unnatural, instances of younger men having a crush on older women is nothing new.

So, what is it that attracts men to women older to them?

In *Dil Chahta Hai,* we saw a down to earth guy like Akshaye Khanna falling in love with Dimple Kapadia, a divorcee, much older to him, while his happy-go-lucky friends Saif and Aamir got attracted to younger girls. The fIlm had a message that Akshay was seeking a friend who could understand his work and his emotions; he had no time for a frivolous relationship.

Ad man Prahlad Kakkar reveals, "I had a relationship with a twenty three year-old woman when I was just sixteen. She told me that she found me cute and that she would teach me all about women. So you see, there was a reversal of roles here. I liked her because she was in control and my mentor."

The awe factor

For young teenage guys, it is nothing but the simple awe of a grown-up woman that attracts them to her. Says Neelesh Kapur, a DU student, "When I was in Class fifth, I was attracted to my Geography teacher. She was just so pretty and used to smell great too. I was just astounded by her beauty; there wasn't anything sexual about it."

Model-turned-actor Milind Soman has been famous for his casanova image. But, the first time he fell in love, he was eleven while the girl was twelve. "She was smart, talented and charismatic and wanted to do things with her life. It was totally one-sided till I was seventeen and we actually started seeing each other. This lasted for two years," recollects Milind.

Maturity

Like the case of Akshaye in *Dil Chahta Hai*, many men find older women more mature and capable of understanding them better. Also, older women are more capable of handling relationships. According to model-turned-actor Zulfi, 'Age doesn't matter if you find a mature woman who can handle the relationship well. Things have changed today. With more and more women working, there aren't many ego hassles between the couple anymore." Zulfi has not dated an older woman but if he could, he would choose Salma Hayek. "She is so beautiful and talented. A mix of Indian and Western looks. She looks hot and acts well and I do not mind that she is older," he adds.

Biologically, women reach their sexual prime in their 30s and men do so in their 20s. So, doesn't that mean that men should always date older women? "Well, a short-term fling can be fun but this certainly cannot be a rule. There is a flip side to the sexual clocks too. While women menopause in their forties, men don't," says a relationship expert.

Is the relationship sustainable?

Yes:

The age difference is not so drastic. Says Kakkar, "With time, a couple either grows. closer to each other or away from each other. And if the age gap is very desparate, then chances of their growing apart are even more."

The emotional security of the partner also counts. Says Garima Roshan, a BPO executive, who broke off with her boyfriend a year back, "Initially, I was very happy with him. I was 28 and he was 17. But I started getting insecure about our future, I feared what would happen when I am forty and he is twenty-nine? He would loose all interest in me!"

And then there is the compatibility factor. "Relationships can be stable when both partners, whatever their relative age, have the same or compatible view of life and what they want from it," says Milind.

No:

The woman carries too much baggage about her past. Along with maturity and sexual experience, an older woman may also come with a lot of baggage about her past relationships. Says Purnima Bakshi, a DU student, "This was evident in *Dil Chahta Hai*. Dimple was too attached to her daughter and was shattered by her earlier relationship. This can cause problems in a new relationship with a younger man. Both have to be terribly mature and emotionally strong to sail through the troubles of this tie."

Courtesy – TOI

Happy Couples

Smell of Success

Will pheromone fragrances help men attract more women ? Atleast that's what the sellers claim.

Pheromones are chemicals naturally given off in small amounts by all men in fresh sweat. The smell of pheromones is quite different from the less attractive smell of body odour, which is caused by skin bacterial breaking down old sweat. And studies suggest that women do find male pheromones sexually attractive - a primitive instinct seen in many animal species. However, quite frankly, physical appearance, body language and personality all play far more important roles in the initial stages of sexual attraction. So while good-smelling pheromones may help when you get up close, you can't rely on them !

The Good, The Bad & The Sexy

On days when you have the headache, and she's all gunge, what do you do ? Never spurn her overtures, she will never let you forget it. But no need to sweat it either, if you can't get an erection—after all, you aren't in the frame of mind for horseplay. What's the solution ? This is where you turn to toys. With a little external aid, she'll not only have her fun, but helping her may also put you right back in the mood. So which ones to go shopping for ? Here's the surprise :

What's Hyped : Rubber Diodes

Those 14" veined monstrosities have nothing on you. They don't move. You have to do all the work. Ditto for cucumbers, bananas and stick deodorants.

What's Hot # 1 : Electronic Toothbrush

Too shy to pick up a vibrator of the phallic kind ? Batty Godson, high priestess of self love, recommends that you buy an electric toothbrush. Saw off one of the brush ends. File and sand paper the end of the plastic remainder to a smooth round contour. Inserted into the electric unit, it serves as a lovely clitoris estimator. The small cylindrical vibrating head - about the size of a little finger - may seem an unlikely candidate, but there is nothing to panic.

What's Hot # 2 : Bathroom Spray

Start outside and rotate the water in a circle around the clitoris, making the temperature older or warmer, for different sensations.

Why do some women fart during sex ? Is it unnatural ? It kind of kills the moment....

Actually, it's quite common, completely natural and a harmless part of sex. There is often a small increase in air pressure in the vagina during sex, and the easiest escape route for the air is around the outside of the penis. This may introduce some unwelcome comedy, but as it's something everyone experiences and does not signify anything untoward, it's probably best to laugh about it rather than get embarrassed. There's no definitive solution, as it's not something that's widely commented on in medical journals ! It is, however, likely that some positions brings this on more than others, so stick to the latter. It's also likely to be more of a problem if you stop and restart during sex.

Read Her Sex Signals

Women carp endlessly about not getting enough foreplay, complain about having to fake orgasms in order to please their mate, but rarely ever do you hear them describe in explicit terms, what exactly they expect you to do, or even what the sexual experience does for them. Which is a pity. Because how are you supposed to know what pleases a woman if she doesn't tell?

Relax. Below is a step-by-step account of everything she feels, thinks, wonders and wants when she's making love to you. It'll show you what you can do to help her enjoy the sexual experience, and in so doing enhance your own pleasure. And finally, it'll uncover the essential truth - that a woman's journey during sex is really nothing like a man's.

This is priceless information, gentlemen.

STEP 1: THE MOOD

What puts a woman in the mood for sex? A factor no man should underemphasize is that making love is as much an emotional event for a woman as it is a physical one. And a big component of that is simply feeling good about herself and your relationship. If life is too hectic lately, eg. she's breast feeding, or if she's feeling bloated, fat or inactive, sex may not enthuse her.

While that may sound a little discouraging, there are a number of things you can do to help put your partner in the mood for love.

One : Concentrate as hard on the friendship part of your relationship as you do on the physical part. If you're intimate in conversation, you can bet she'll be intimate in bed. In one survey, women who felt especially close to their mates reported having excellent sex lives—no matter how they felt about their own bodies.

Two : Constantly tell her how great she is. Compliment. Give her a lustful look. Whisper your wicked desires into her ears. Get her to buy the idea that she's lustworthy, and she'll aim to prove it to you.

STEP 2: THE AROUSAL

If you've succeeded in getting her in the mood, she'll now want to see some action to kickstart her libido, probably exhibit a strong desire to be kissed and kissed well.

You probably already know that a woman's lips, tongue and mouth are some of the most erogenous zones of her body. Stimulating them properly can actually arouse her down below. But kissing is also a way of communicating. A well-timed, well-executed lip lock helps give a woman the emotional closeness she's looking for.

But what's the right way to kiss her? First of all, take your time. If you pay attention to kissing well instead of rushing passionately on (hint: don't just stick your tongue down her mouth, chew, lick her lips), you'll be at second base before you know it. Vary the pressure, the duration, the location of your lips and keep your hands busy - grab her hair, her bottom.

Now you may be focusing on her lips, but it's only a matter of moments before her whole body will react. Her breathing, heart rate and blood pressure will begin to increase, her nipples will become erect and her areolae will swell.

Within 15 to 20 seconds of arousal, her vagina will start to moisten. Maybe most important, she'll start to feel turned on all over her body.

The sensitivity of a woman's entire body cannot be overemphasized. While the key to a man's sexual pleasure lies between his legs, women are less focused on the genitals and more aware of other parts of their bodies. The late sex researcher Alfred Kinsey found some women who were capable of reaching orgasm simply by having their eyebrows stroked, their earlobes kissed or some pressure applied to their teeth.

What does this mean for you? Well, start exploring. Find a brave new world. If you've already struck the usual erogenous zones like the breasts, invent some new ones. The unexpected sensation is what you're after here, and you just might ambush her into orgasm.

One warning at this stage: While it's true that direct stimulation of the clitoris—the little pink area above the woman's vagina - is the key to most women's climaxing, don't pounce too quickly. As a woman becomes more and more aroused, the clitoris will swell, producing a sort of erection. But her erection takes longer than yours does to develop, and any direct contact before that point can be painful.

STEP 3 : THE GATHERING MOMENTUM

By now her skin will be flushed, her eyes wide and pupils dilated. But there are other signs of sexual readiness.

Swelling Breasts

You already know that an erect nipple is a good sign, but according to pioneering sex researchers Masters and Johnson, a woman's entire breast can swell as much as 25 per cent during arousal. In addition, her areolas will darken.

Swollen Labia

When a woman becomes very aroused, her vaginal lips (labia) swell slightly and begin to move away from their usual position covering the opening of the vagina.

Once you've noticed these signs, it's time to stimulate her down there, either with your hands or your lips.

All women have different preferences during oral sex, so the best advice is to experiment: Use both sides of your tongue, for example, or let your tongue go soft in such a way that you'd slur your words if you tried to speak. While you work, ask her to provide a play-by play of what she's feeling.

There's one problem with oral sex, however. No matter what's going on in a woman's body, in her head she might be feeling insecure about how she smells or tastes down there. A simple reassurance from you that the neighbourhood is fine - "You taste so good" - should nip that in the bud, as it were. Many women are also troubled off by the taste of their own vaginal juices, so don't rush to kiss her immediately afterward.

Generally speaking, the happy recipient of oral sex is willing to reciprocate for her man. The operative word is 'generally' because the act itself isn't physically sensational for a woman. Her lips can dry out quickly and chafe, she may gag. (A quick shower before sex does wonders.)

Give her verbal reinforcement, kind words, feedback to keep her going. Most important, be a gentleman: This act needs to be her idea and her pleasure. No coercion, no pushing.

With this in mind, oral sex can actually be a major turn-on for your partner. In her head she's satisfying her fantasy role of a siren.

STEP 4: THE PLUNGE

This is what you've been waiting for.

The moment of penetration can be physically pleasant for a woman, but, alas, the sensation doesn't last long. After a couple of minutes, the initial thrill of being entered wears off and penetration turns into intercourse. Because the clitoris isn't normally stimulated during missionary-position sex, and

because there are few nerve endings in the rear two thirds of the vagina, most women don't get much pleasure from this physically, especially if you pump away mindlessly.

What to do about it? Kissing or breast touching can help, but the best solution may be to try a different position. Woman-on-top is classic for letting her grind to orgasm but side-by-side or rear-entry sex, both of which allow her to stimulate herself while you're inside her, are also effective.

Yet another option: Pay attention to your own thrusting technique. In their book *The Multi-Orgasmic Man*, authors Mantak Chia and Douglas Arava suggest an ancient Oriental pattern of nine shallow thrusts. followed by one deep one. Try it, it might just work, especially given the fact that the majority of a woman's nerve endings are in the front of the vagina.

Lastly, don't let the act of intercourse go on for too long; your partner will simply get tired and her mind will start to wander. And that's the last effect you want to create.

STEP 5: THE VERGE

All is going according to plan. She's on the verge of orgasm.

What does it feel like for her? For a woman, the pre-orgasm sensation is otherworldly, ethereal. (No wonder its often called peaking.)

But just because a woman reaches the edge doesn't mean she's going to have an orgasm. Unlike men, women don't experience the unrelenting, inevitable line drive toward orgasm. It's more of a roundabout path. She may get close, then backslide, even have to fantasize to push herself over the edge.

If your partner doesn't have an orgasm, the reason might be purely physical, or it might be that she's feeling too much pressure (from you) to have one.

To avoid that, feel free to focus on your own pleasure, but make sure she knows how good it feels to be inside her.

Getting her thinking about you will stop her thinking about herself, and that might be all she needs to let it happen.

Of course, there are times when a woman would just as soon forget the whole thing. When your partner says it's okay not to have an orgasm once in a while, she means it. If you really want to up her odds, invest in that magic wand, the vibrator.

STEP 6: THE CLIMAX

The most important thing to know about a woman's orgasm is this: she screams during the middle of it, she's faking. Here's why: While climaxing, it's nearly impossible to exhale. The female orgasm is not an explosion of endorphins and genital juices. It's an implosion. She'll draw her breath, tighten her muscles, suck every scrap of energy and sensation into the tiny nut core of her being and then give way exquisitely, to the flow of goodness spreading up her chest and down her legs.

STEP 7: THE AFTER GLOW

This may be where you find the most variation in style. Although what women experience physically after orgasm is the same across the board the genitals return to their normal state, and breathing and heart rates slow to normal—emotionally and psychologically no two women are alike. Some feel huggy and affectionate; others want to talk about life; others just wonder what's on HBO.

The best advice? Seal the emotional bond with a kiss, a compliment, a final squeeze. By the time you're in your postcoital snooze, she'll still be happily awake, thinking of you as a man who really made a connection.

Last Forever in Bed

How to keep sex alive and kicking through the years without pills and potions

- Remember disuse, not use, leads to atrophy of your sexual organs.
- Regular sex will increase your production of testosterone.
- So will exercise, especially weight training. Exercise has the aadditional benefit of helping you to lose weight, look better, and get your ciruclation and libido going.
- Think of sex as a means of closeness, appreciation and tenderness.
- Accept that older nervous systems and tissues resulting slower arousals and weaker erection response; so tone down your expectations.
- Devote more time to foreplay or make foreplay an alternative to actual intercouse.
- Focus on pleasure not performance.
- Have sex in the morning when you have more energy.
- Start a meaningful relationship with your partner, or find a new love if you are single. Experiment into locations, massages, showers. Titillating books and movies.
- Eat well balanced meals with less saturated fats that

can clog up your blood vessels and slow down your responses.

- Cut down on smoking and drinking.
- Think positively of all the things that you have achieved and hope to achieve.
- Even if you do not get an erection bring your partner to orgasm.
- Don't be embarrassed to ask your doctor to suggest custom-made sex gizmos to suit your medical condition.

To get top result from Viagra

- Consult your doctor, not your chemist before you start.
- Take the pill 2 hours after a modrate meal. A full stomach delays absorption.
- Attempts sex after one or two hours.
- Sexual stimulation is necessary to strengthen and amplify your erection.
- If not satisfied ask your doctor for a higher dose.

The doctor must evaluate lipid levels and the prostate before starting, because testosterone supplements may aggravate existing prostate cancer, can (ironically) cause gynecomastia (enlarged breasts) in some; precipitate or worsen sleep apnoea; and increase risk of heart disease.

If a low testosterone level is not the only determinant in impotence, what else is ?

Impotence or Erectile Dysfunction is the persistent inability of a man to achieve and maintain an erection strong enough for penetrative sex. A lot many factors go into an erection. Like

- the brain, which has a fine network of erogenous stimuli.
- the nerves, which pass messages from the brain to the penis.

• the blood vessels in the penis.

An erection occurs when the arteries supplying the penis dilate, thus increasing the blood flow to it.

70% of impotence cases are caused by a noxious brew of psychological causes, such as fear of age, inhibitions, ignorance, fear, stress, boredom, embarrassment, poor body image, depression, traumatic sexual escapades, pressure to perform, unrealistic expectations, performance anxiety and more.

30% suffer from physical causes where the blood vessels of the penis are damaged because of diabetes, hypertension, high cholesterol, spinal injury, excessive drinking and smoking. Contrary to public opinion, prescribed drugs such as anti-hypertensives and antidepressants account for only 100/6 of these and only 1% are caused by hormonal imbalances.

40% of men at 40 have mild erectile dysfunctions.

70% of men at 70 have severe erectile dysfunction.

How can you slot the problem?

It is psychological if :

- you wake up with an erection
- you can masturbate perfectly well
- you have had satisfactory penetrative intercourse
- your problem occurred suddenly

It is physical if :

- your erection is feeble and does not strengthen even while you sleep, wake up or masturbate
- you try and try but do not succeed
- the onset comes gradually, insidiously

Is impotence linked to heart disease?

If you have puffed arteries in your penis it is likely that the blood vessels of your heart are unhealthy. So impotence can be a sign that a cardiogram is overdue.

If testosterone replacement is not an option, what are the treatment choices available for impotence?

There are injections, implants, pumps. Surgery is an option for some. And then of course there's Viagra.

Tell us how this wonder pill works.

Sildenafil Citrate, famous as Viagra, has spawned a clutch of cheaper, equally efficacious Indian clones, from Silagra to Penegra.

It blocks the enzyme E-phospho-diesterase Type V in the penis so that the penile blood vessels open out within an hour, helped by stimulation. It-works for six to 8 hours.

It is suitable for men who have'a normal blood supply to the penis but cannot become dilated because of diabetes, hypertension, nerve damage, liver damage, performance anxiety and is 70% to 75% effective. What's more, it can be taken privately. 20% of users report minor symptoms - congestion of the nose and eyes, acidity, heaviness of the head - which are not life threatening. It is only dangerous for those on nitrates for Coronary Heart Disease, because the interaction can reduce blood pressure drastically. However it does not trigger heart attacks for any other reason.

So how can older men keep smiling?

By calling their condition impotence not andropause. Because impotence can be treated. Counselling, procedures, devices and drugs mean that men no longer have to sacrifice sexuality to age.

Sex on Drugs

Viagra has sired a slew of potent remedies that promise better and better performance in bed.

- Tadalafil (Cialis), makes for more spontaneity as it works for upto 36 hours, which is why it is nicknamed the Weekened Pill - you can take it a Friday night and the effect lasts till Sunday.
- Vardenafil, has been tested on Indian patients very successfully, is more potent than Sildenafil, but is not yet available in India.
- And then there's the brand new drug for permature ejaculation all set to hit the market. Dapoxetine, originally an antidepressant, may not only make a man last longer in bed but also increase sexual stamina more than threefold.

Myths of the Youngsters

Before entering into the vast field of sex, let us dispel certain myths and unreasoned, baseless and unfounded notions about certain sex matters as also about sex organs. Entire description will revolve around martial coitus and marital sex, even though scattered reference to other topics, may be found here and there.

Length of Penis

It is often a male gender worry. Some people think that by having a lengthy penis they can get more sexual pleasure during coition and that their partner would also get sexually 'worked up' or excited as, according to him (the male), she loves husbands / men who have long penis. Men also nurture an idea that their spouse prefers the persons who have long and hard penis. But, certain women also are afraid that by pushing the lengthy penis in their vaginas, their male partners will rip their vaginas apart.

Actually speaking, length of a penis must not cause any sort of inferiority complex or any fear in the minds of either sex. It is not the length that matters, but what matters is as to how long and how best a man can satisfy his spouse. Short length of male organ should be no cause of concern for any male. Certain men, even when they have long penis do ejaculate earlier and thus fail to satisfy their sexually aroused women. On the contrary some men, even with not lengthy penis, are not found inferior in sexually satisfying their women. The women are not concerned with the penile length, they are concerned, of course, as to how best their men can quench their sexual thirst to achieve orgasm. Length of penis is a mere psychological phobia which must be dispelled as soon as possible.

When a penis is 'placcid' (or in Non-erect position) is usually is 3" long or so, and 4" or so from base to tip. In normal erectile position length of a penis would be around $6\frac{1}{2}$" or so, with slight variations. So, it is rather immaterial as to how long penis a person has. What, in fact matters and should matter as to how and in what way, and, above all, how long can a man hold his ecstasy.

A word of caution for the ladies. They should never demoralise their husbands or ridicule them, belittle them or compare them with other persons, as far as length of penis is concerned, who have got longer penis. The poor fellow would be deeply hurt, and may even become impotent. For the male to view his penis in a mirror or in a bath room would relieve, reassure and also satisfy his ego and thus his inferiority complex would vanish. Moreover, length of a penis has no relation with virility and sex performance of a man.

Never let the penile size be a hurdle in the enjoyment of sexual act, rather concentrate your attention, on other new aspects of love play.

Vaginal Size and Depth

Young married ladies are scared to approach or be approached by their husbands for the sheer fear that entry of penis would rip apart their vaginas. As already explained, the soft tissues in the vagina are so spongy, soft and flexible that they can accommodate any kind of male organ. The male also shouldn't have any such misgiving either. If the woman is properly excited during pre-coital play (or foreplay) the' vagina, gets lubricated. Simple point to keep in mind is that if a woman can expel the baby from her vagina then where does the size of a male organ stand? Vagina is like a roomy passage, which extends upwards and backwards several inches with soft, well bolstered comfortable walls and the pleasurable 'dewy secretion' that lubricates the opening, makes it easy to slip out and slip in. This love juice is generated by the vaginal walls which pour the secretion ahead. According to Masters and Johnson, within 30 seconds the woman's vagina is moist enough to allow entry of male penis. Lubrication and muscular relaxation will facilitate male organ entry. So, the real job is done by the lubricating vagina juice. Actually a lubricated vagina is indicative of its readiness to accept entry of male organ.

The best way for a woman to keep her vaginal muscles in perfect humour is to do exercise with vaginal muscles by way of expansion and contraction. This process would also strengthen the muscles and tighten them also.

Sex Facts & Fallacies

True Lies

Common wisdom says that masturbation is emasculating, and sex before a big race is a no-no. Now find out the truth about these legends.

Common Wisdom

Men reach their sexual peak at 18, and women reach theirs at 28.

Fact With regard to both sexes' supply of sexual hormones, at least, this is true. Testosterone peaks at age 18 in men; womens estrogen hits its higher point in the mid-20s. But peak hormones don't mean peak sexual performance.

Common Wisdom : Semen is all protein.

Fallacy : Semen is mostly fruit sugar (fructose) and

enzymes—not protein.

Common Wisdom : Masturbation yields the strongest orgasm.

Fact - But it's not a hard-and-fast rule, as it were. It depends on the individual. For some it does, but for others, there's nothing that beats pleasure of intercourse.

Common Wisdom

Having sex before an important event—the big race, the critical presentation—can ruin your performance in the event.

Fallacy

Swiss researchers performed stress tests on people 2 and 10 hours after the subjects has had sex, and found that by 10 hours, the participants were fully recovered. There was only a small dip in performance 2 hours after sex.

Q-A On Male Sexuality

What is premature ejaculation ?

This is one of the most common sexual disorders, perhaps as common as the common cold. Generally, "climaxing" before one wants to is considered as "premature ejaculation". This term confuses orgasm with ejaculation. This is early orgasmic response wherein an individual experience orgasm earlier than his idealized expectation.

What are the causes of premature ejaculation ?

The causes may be primary, wherein the disorder exists from the beginning, or secondary, wherein it occurs subsequent to a prior normal function. The causes are illustrated as follows :

Situations	Constitutional
(usually primary)	(usually secondary)
Anxiety	Diabetes mellitus
Sexual inexperience	Neurological disorders
Deterioration of relationship	Genito-urinary pathology
Prolonged abstinence	
Victimization by partner	
Unrealistic expectation from self / partner.	

What is phimosis ?

Inability to retract the foreskin (prepuce) due to adhesions between the foreskin and the glans penis is called phimosis. It may lead to pain, frenulum tear or paraphimosis during intercourse and also predisposes the individual to recurrent infections. it can be prevent by good local hygience and can be easily cured by circumcision.

What is a penile implant ?

A penile implant is a mechanical device used in cases of erectile dysfunction. It is implanted into the penis and is not an artificial penis. There are two varieties of penile implants. One is the semi-rigid implant and the other is the inflatable implant (three-part implant). The details are tabulated as follows -

Semi--rigid	Inflatable	
Cost	Less	More
Appearance	Always erect	Under your control
Comfort	Less	More
Consistency (Hardness)	Fixed	Adjustable
Compilcations	Less	More
Surgery	Less time and skill	More time and skill

Is it advisable to use a rubber band or a cloth strip around the penis in cases of impotence ?

No, such a practice is extremely dangerous, as instances of gangrene have been reported in such cases.

What about orgasm and ejaculation after implant surgery?

The quality and quantity of orgasm and ejaculation remain unaffected by the surgery, i.e., the patient will experience an orgasm and will have an ejaculation as he used to have prior to the surgery.

What are the common causes of pain in an erect penis ?

Phimosis, paraphimosis, local injuries, ulcers, and urethral and prostatic inflammation are known to cause pain on erection. At times in Peyronie's disease or fibrous cavernositis, pain on erection may be a common symptom. Priapism is another condition in which there is prolonged painful erection.

At times, just following an erection or prior to ejaculation, a drop or two of a sticky transparent fluid oozes out from the penis. Is this normal ?

Yes. In such situations, the fluid which comes out is the secretion of Cowper's glands or bulbourethra glands. When one encounters a sexual situation, there is secretion (akin to salivation) from the cowper's glands.

Can this fluid cause pregnancy ?

No

Is the penis usually inclined towards the left ?

Yes, this is true for a majority of men. This is so perhaps because the left testis is lower than the right. Therefore, while wearing their undergarments, most when adjust their penis on the left side as more space exists on the left as compared to the right.

Does a slight curvature of the penis lead to any difficulty in penetration ?

No. A slight curvature of the penis, either to the left or to the right, is common and does not affect the ability to penetrate at all.

Is it a fact that a woman must bleed at the first attempt at sexual intercourse ?

No. Such bleeding usually occurs due to the rupture of the hymen in virgins. However, the hymen may be absent from birth or might rupture while playing games, doing exercises or using tampons. Hence, a woman may not bleed during the first sexual intercourse though she is a virgin. I have seen many marriages on the rocks because of this misconception. It is a matter of a big issue over a small tissue !

Do men have a greater sex drive than women ?

The sexual urge depends on the individual's sexuality and a greater sex drive is not the prerogative of either sex !

What are sleep emission ? Are they normal ?

Sleep emissions or "nightfalls" represent a normal physiological phenomenon. Semen is being secreted continuously by the genital apparatus ; it has to be expelled by some means. If one does not have sex or does not masturbate either, semen gets expelled in the form of sleep emission. The situation is akin to a glass full of water to which you add more water with the logical result that it overflows.

What is masturbation ?

Masturbation is self-stimulation of the genitals for pleasure, which may or may not be pursued to the point of orgasm.

How do men masturbate ?

For men, the most common method is to hold the penis with the hand, so as to encircle it in the palm and produce friction by to-and-from movements, often till orgasm and ejaculation are reached. Variation such as mimicking coital movements against bedclothes, a pillow, pressing against some objects are also common.

What is the "normal standard time" for an intercourse ?

There is no "normal standard time" for an intercourse. It depends upon the partners. Intercourse may be continued till it is mutually satisfying. A prolonged intercourse does not necessarily give more pleasure. This is a myth. What is important is not how long, but how satisfying !

How often should a couple have sexual intercourse ?

Sexual intercourse is the means to an end, the end being pleasure. Therefore, a couple can have intercourse as often as it pleases them. It is a pleasure to be shared between the partners and there is no need to keep a tally. "Frequent" or "normal" depends upon the individual couple. The best thing to do is to forget the number game and indulge as often as it is mutually pleasurable and satisfying. What is important is the quality and not the quality.

Is frequent intercourse harmful ?

Present medical knowledge acknowledges the fact that as long as intercourse occurs among accepting partners and is not associated with physical trauma of irritation, the act itself is not harmful, irrespective of its frequency.

Is testicular self-examination (TSE) necessary for an adult male ?

Yes. Every adult male should perform the TSE every month. If testicular malignancy is diagnosed early, it can be cured completely. **What are the symptoms and signs of testicular tumours?**

The first sign of testicular malignancy is usually a slight enlargement of one of the testes and a change is consistency. Pain may be absent but often there is a dull ache in the lower abdomen and groin together with a dragging sensation and heaviness.

How does one perform the TSE ?

The TSE involves a simple, three-minute monthly self-examination. The best time is after a warm bath or shower, when the scrotal skin is the most relaxed. The following are the simple steps for an effective TSE :

- Do the TSE first on one testicle, then on the other.
- Use both hands to examine each testicle.
- Place your fingers behind your testicle, with the thumb in the front.
- Roll each testicle gently between the thumb and fingers of both hands. Most likely, the testicles will feel smooth and spongy if they are completely normal. But if your feel any hard lumps or nodules on the front or side of the testicles, you must see your doctor promptly.

The TSE is a healthy habit and it should be practised regularly, every month.

Q-A On Female Sexuality

Does pre-menstrual tension affect sexuality ?

Yes, it does. Women tend to become irritable with associated symptoms such as nausea, backache and breast tenderness. There is a feeling of discomfort in the pelvic region and, at times, there may be emotional disturbances and varying degrees of depression. In some women, however, it is found that the sex drive is enhanced, perhaps resulting from increased pelvic congestion, insufficient to cause discomfort but sufficient to cause intense pelvic awareness.

Do oral contraceptive pills prevent pre menstrual tension?

Yes, oral contraceptive pills do relieve premenstrual tension in about 50 percent and painful periods, i.e., dysmenorrhoea, in 90 percent of the women.

Can the breast size be increased ?

Certain exercises can help develop the pectoralis major muscles which would add a little bulk to the chest (but not to the breast themselves) and this may help increase the apparent breast size. Plastic surgery (silicone implant) may also prove beneficial. However, one needs to understand the risks involved before undergoing surgery.

Does disparity in breast size require treatment ?

Disparity in the size of the breasts may be due to various reasons—physiological and pathological. Disparity due to any pathological cause must be thoroughly investigated and treated. For physiological disparity, no treatment, other than counselling and reassurance, is required. For cosmetic reasons, if the difference is minor, padding the brassiere cup of the smaller beat would suffice. If the difference in size or contour is gross, then an enhancement / enlargement mammoplasty of the smaller breast or a reduction mammoplasty of the larger one may be carried out after evaluating each case on individual merit.

Does hair on the breast suggest any pathology ?

It is not uncommon for a woman to have a few hair around the aureola of the breast which does not need any treatment. However, they may be removed by electrolysis by a qualified person, if one desires.

Is it necessary to stimulate the clitoris during sexual intercourse ?

Some women report that they get enough clitoral stimulation during normal sexual intercourse. Some prefer gentle stimulation along with a little pressure. For some women, intercourse is enough to reach a climax, while for others additional clitoral stimulation is essential.

What is the G-spot and how can one stimulate it ?

The G-spot, or the Grafenberg spot, is an area of increased sensitivity with maximum potential for arousal. It is located on the anterior vaginal wall about two inches from the vaginal opening. After sliding the fingers and with forward, backward or side to side movement, the female will be able to pinpoint the spot where she experiences increased sensitivity. With increased stimulation, the G-spot swells like a nodule, and becomes firm. Simultaneous clitoral stimulation can enhance sexual pleasure.

[Some females enjoy talks of sex, intecourse etc. during foreplay to get excitement prior to start intercourse].

What is the most common female sexual problem ?

Painful sexual intercourse or inadequate sexual arousal is the most common sexual problem in females.

Note : Painful sexual intercourse need not always be

due to inadequate sexual arousal. It can exist as an independent entity.

What could be the cause of excessive vaginal lubrication during sexual intercourse?

Physiologically, lubrication occurs in the vaginal lubrication during sexual arousal. This could increase in certain conditions of heightened sexual excitement and vaginal infection or allergy. The best course is to find the cause and treat it. At times, a small dose of an antihistamine may prove useful.

Do women have different degrees of lubrication ?

Yes, women differ in the amount of vaginal lubrication produced. Even in the same woman, the lubrication may different from time to time and it depends upon the intensity of stimulation provided. There are also several causes of reduced levels of lubrication as inadeuate sexual arousal, local vaginal infection and hormonal imbalances. Adequate vaginal lubrication is essential for pain free penetration.

Partners need to communicate about their likes and dislikes. They may also need to increase the time of foreplay. Psychological stimulation such as erotic talk, fantasizing, reading and viewing erotic material may also prove useful. These stimulants will help increase arousal and hence will aid vaginal lubrication.

Can a virgin become pregnant ?

Yes, if the sperms are deposited near the vulva, they may pass through the small pores of an intact hymen and may travel up through the vagina and uterus and fertilize the ovum, resulting in pregnancy.

Is sex safe during pregnancy ?

Usually, a healthy woman can safely indulge in sexual activity during pregnancy. However, coitus should be avoided if there is a pain and / or bleeding at any stage. If the woman has aborted in the first three months in the past, coitus during the first trimester should be avoided. In the second trimester coitus is contraindicated if the woman has a history of "habitual abortion" because the certival os, i.e., the mouth of the uerus is incompetent to hold the foetus. In the last trimester, i.e., from the seventh month to labour, one may safely indulge in sexual activity till the day of delivery by adorning the position so as to ensure that the direct weight does not fall on the foetus.

It must be understood that whenever, because of any reason, intercourse is forbidden during pregnancy, the woman must avoid reaching orgasm by any other means including masturbation. The contraction of the uterus following masturbation are far more intense as compared to those of normal sexual intercourse.

An obstetrician may be consulted regarding the indulgence in sexual activity during pregnancy as each case needs to be evaluated individually.

Are alcohol and smoking safe during pregnancy ?

No, both alcohol and smoking are unsafe during pregnancy as they may lead to intrauterine growth retardation and foetal malformation.

When can a woman resume sexual intercourse after delivery ?

One should not indulge in sexual intercourse :

(1) If the episiotomy scar (the cut made to ease the birth of the baby) has not healed properly.

(2) If there is bleeding from vagina.

Usually, after three weeks of delivery, a woman can comfortably resume sexual activity.

Is episiotomy necessary during normal delivery ?

Episiotomy facilitates delivery of the foetal head and prevents uncontrolled vaginal and perennial tears. Episiotomy is not mandatory, but it plays a protective role.

After pregnancy, many times, couples report that they do not experience the pleasure that they used to. Can this be helped ?

After normal delivery often vaginal walls become lax and the penovaginal contact reduces. Thus some people do report less pleasure. This can be helped, while during the episiotomy, the obsterician should take one or more stitches, known as "husband's stitch", to ensure adequate apposition which help in increasing the penovaginal contact, thus giving more pleasure.

What is the most common cause of a lax vagina ? How can it be prevented ?

This may occur following childbirth. It can be best prevented by proper management of labour with perineal support and prenatal exercises.

What is the treatment for a lax vagina ?

A lax vagina can benefit from Kagel's exercises. It involves contraction of the perineal muscles - a phenomenon akin to holding the urine and releasing it. Twenty such contractions and relaxations, three times a day, may help increase the muscle tone. If this does not work, one may consider vaginal reconstructive surgery.

What conditions can make a woman frigid ?

Distraction, disturbed interpersonal relationships, anti-hypertensive drugs, tranquillizers, sedatives, hypnotise and sometimes oral contraceptives can lead to a decline in sexual desire. Pain at the time of coitus, whether due to vaginitis, pelvic infection or abnormal uterine positions, may lead to frigidity of sudden onset.

What is female circumcisions ?

It is a barbaric custom of female genital mutilation. In its most disfiguring form - the Pharonic circumcision practised in Sudan and Kenya - it involves cutting off of the clitoris, labia major and labia minor followed by close apposition of the tissue that remains, leaving only a tiny hole at the bottom for the passage of urine. This severe local mutilation make sex a painful encounter. In its mildest form, it involves excision of the clitoris or the clitoral hood alone. Such circumcision is performed due to the misconception* that unless it is performed a woman will become overtly promiscuous.

Do women masturbate ? How ?

Yes, women do masturbate. The usual method is by rubbing a finger on the clitoris. The female anatomy permits considerable variations such as thigh rubbing, rubbing clothing between the thighs, and so on.

Do women ejaculate ?

Some women do report squirting of fluid at the time of orgasm, but this is rare. Whether this can be called female ejaculation is controversial.

Is there a phenomenon in women akin to wet dreams in men ?

Yes, women too can have erotic dreams and become aroused and lubricated during sleep. Sometimes, she can even have an orgasm. As there is no ejaculation it is not really a wet dream.

What are women's misunderstandings about men's sexuality which may lead to sexual dysfunctions ?

Often, when a man is a premature ejaculator, many women may consider him a poor lover or the woman may make an attempt to reach orgasm early. At times, this kind of thinking leads to a shortening of the period of intimacy. In cases of retarded ejaculation, where there is a delay in reaching orgasm, the woman starts getting a feeling that her partner does not love her or she is not attractive to him any more, which may disturb the intimate relationship. Also, most women consider it improper to actively participate in intercourse and prefer to remain completely passive or only minimally responsive, leaving the onus on the male who is now under pressure to perform. This may create a situation anxiety that may impair his response and performance. Even if the male is able to perform properly in these circumstances, the minimal or deliberately subdued response of his partner due to traditional misconceptions will leave him with the fleeing that the encounter has not been mutually satisfying. If this occurs repeatedly, it instils a sense of inadequacy and frustration in him that may affect his performance and his sex drive may decline.

How should a physician deal with a sexual problem ?

After an adequate history taking, the physician should try to determine exactly where the problem lies; i.e., misconceptions, unrealistic expectation, disturbed interpersonal relationships or hostility towards a partner. The physician should counsel the couple as a unit, clarify and explain the situation to them and clean misconceptions. He may offer specific therapy if and when the situation demands.

What are the psychological sequelae of a rape case ?

The psychological trauma experienced in a rape victim often exceeds the physical trauma. The affected individual loses her sense of self-confidence and self-esteem and becomes increasingly aware of her vulnerability. She developed negative attitudes towards sex. This will affect her response and performance in subsequence sexual encounters. Some victims avoid sexual intimacy and even if they do indulge, often they tend to recreate and relive the traumatic experience and are unable to continue the encounter. Sometimes, the society also considers the victim as promiscuous, who has probably invited the tragedy upon herself. She also becomes the object of the unsolicited attention of males looking for a casual temporary relationship. This could result in further loss of self-esteem and is psychologically detrimental.

Why and how should one perform breast self-examination?

Almost all breast malignancies are first detected by the women themselves. Detection of breast cancer in the early stages, when it is localized, is of paramount importance, because if treated early, the disease can be cured completely. Hence, the importance of self examination of the breasts, monthly, as a routine healthy habit, to be practised by all women above the age of 20 years should be emphasized. It should be performed at about the same time every month, just after the monthly period, when breast is least likely to be nodular. One must look for any changes since the last time the breasts were examined.

The examination may be performed as follows, examining one breast at a time, first inspecting and then palpating the breast.

Inspection

1. Start by sitting or standing in front of a mirror, with arms relaxed at the sides. Look for a change in the size or the shape of the breast, puckering or dimpling of the skin, and any discharge from or change in, the nipple.
2. Next, look for exactly the same things, after raising both arms over the head.

The inspection is now complete and one may proceed to palpation of the breast looking for any lump or thickening.

Palpation

1. Lie down and put a pillow under the left shoulder, with the left hand under the head. Using the fingers of the right hand, held together and flat, press gently but firmly with small circular movements, to feel the upper inner quarter of the left beast, starting at the breast bone and going outward will you reach the nipple line. Feel the region around the nipple.
2. Similarly examine the lower inner part of the left breast. In this region, a ridge of firm tissue may be felt, which is normal.
3. Now, bringing the hand down to the side, still using the fingers, feel under the armpit.
4. After this, examine the upper outer quarter of the breast, from the nipple line to where your arm is resting, in a similar manner.
5. Lastly, with the same gentle pressure examine the lower outer quarter of the breast, starting from the outer part and going to the nipple.

Repeat the same procedure on the right side completing the examination of the breast.

Thus, one broadly looks for a lump, change in the size or shape, puckering, dimpling or any other skin lesion over the breast and any change or discharge from the nipple.

If any abnormality is detected, do not be alarmed, as all lumps or other changes are not cancerous. However, it is the best to consult a doctor for a complete and proper evaluation of the condition. Breast cancer is curable and an early diagnosis can make all the difference with respect to the prognosis of a given case. Self-examination of the breasts for early detection of malignancy must be developed as a healthy habit and should be continued lifelong.

Mostly Asked Q–A

Here are some questions, which are asked mostly by youngesters.

My grilfriend is into light bondage and pain. We haven't started having sex yet, and from the outset this has been a "different" type of relationship for her. The problem is twofold. Firstly I'm not into 'painful' sex and I can't stand listening to her talk about how much she enjoys kinky sex. So what do I do? I think I'm falling in love with this girl and don't want to end my relationship.

Dude, this relationship is going to end if you don't get a grip on your insecurities. While you have every right not to listen to her whorish war stories, you don't have the right to judge her for them. The next time she starts going into too much detail, politely tell her to shut up. As one-half of a couple who hasn't even had sex yet, it seems like you're doing a lot of worrying in advance. Not only is it unproductive, it's unnecessary. I know you feel strongly about the bondage thing, but I'm just going to throw this one out there, say never. Contrary to popular belief, the most creative, kinky sex doesn't happen the first few times you sleep together. It happens only after a couple has been together for a while and they trust each other enough to let loose their inner deviant. Take it slow, take it easy, and try to relax.

My husband does not trust me. Although he hid his past relationships, it's all out in the open now. He has finally admitted that he was into two other relationships which broke. He feels that I cannot be trusted because I have not been sincere which made him search for solace somewhere else. I have been 100 per cent faithful to him. Our marriage fell apart six months ago when I caught him breaking into my e-mail, reading every things and anything he could find. Please help.

When tow people get married, they become one. You should now concentrate on what is left of the relationship and try to make things work if they have not reached that breaking point. I do think you are being too hard on him and should let him snoop to his heart's content. When you love someone, you have to do everything in your power to ensure that they are secure with your love, especially since you know that he has been hurt before and has trust issues. There is not a single individual who doesn't come into marriage without some baggage. I think that the future success of your marriage is going to depend on whether you accept that we all have hang-ups based on our upbringing and experiences. Of course, you had nothing to do with his present issues, but that doesn't mean you can't help him heal. I think you can build a wonderful life if you can decide that your life will now become an open book to your husband and live with the motto, what's mine is yours. Get over his past and move on with life.

My husband, aged 33, is taking a course of psychotropic medicines for last one and half months. The initial days of our conjugal relationship were absolutely fine (we were married just a few months ago). But of late he is suffering from anorgasmia (though he gets it by other kinds of stimulation like manual but not during intercourse). Now my queries are as follows :-

1) Is it the side effect of the medicine ?
2) Will he be okay in due course of time when the medicine is stopped ?

3) Is there any way to get back to our normal sex life while he's on medication ?

I fear for the days when we both will want to have a baby. I will be immensely grateful if you throw some light on this.

Dr. replies : The problem of anorgasmia that your husband is experiencing is a well known side-effect of the medication he is taking. He will return to normal when the medication is stopped.

Meanwhile, since he can reach an orgasm when stimulated manually you can try the following strategy to regain a normal sexual life while on medication : Stimulate him manually till he is close to orgasm and then have intercourse. This may help him to reach orgasm during intercourse.

I am a 20-year girl. Since the last 2 months, I have been attempting sex, but whenever he tries to enter there is terrible pain in the vagina. This happened 3 times and caused us to cease the activity.

Thereafter I noticed a yellow-white discharge for a few days. This time I had a little bleeding along with discharge, followed by blood tinged discharge for a few days.

I also have a tendency to bleed excessively during periods and suffer from dysmenorrhoea and sometimes menorrhagia. (I take Spasmo Proxivon once a month for dysmenarrhoea.)

Is it just fear or do I actually have some problem? I am worried and scared.

Please help.

You are normal and, like others of your age, badly in need of sex education. Perhaps you and your fience can jointly consult a sex therapist for advise. If fear is dominant in your mind, it may make things easier if the two of you decide to wait till after marriage, Then sex may be partaken in a more relaxed fashion and made more enjoyable.

The little bleeding could possibly be due to the hymen being split. Regarding the pain, perhaps you could invest in a tube of Xylocalne 2% gel and apply a tiny bit around the vaginal opening. After 15 minutes you will experience no pain. A finger may be inserted to test for lubrication. During intercourse keep your legs well flexed and over the abdomen, in opposition to your partner, who will be kneeling in between.

Regarding your other problems you should check with your gynaec. No need to get worried as the problem can be easily solved.

I am 44 years old, married 17 years ago; my wife is 40 years old. We have 2 sons. In the beginning of our married life, my wife did have some hesitation regarding sexual activities whereas I was much interested. So it used to be a one-sided affair, which was very disappointing to me. (Before mariage I used to masturbate very often.) As she gradually understood the esseence of sex, we started having a good time. But then I started experiencing my premature ejaculation. Sometimes within 2-3 seconds of penetration, ejaculation would take place, peaving her, and even me, disappointed. This happened almost 90% of the time. We used to have sex once in a week / fortnight and everytime we would end up in disappointment.

After reading various magazines, I tried all the restraint methods advised. Though somewhat helpful, the pleasure did not last long. Even before my wife got warmed up, I would ejaculate. And now, to add to our miseries, I have developed a problem with arousal as well.

Sometimes, even after a long period of foreplay, there is no erection and even if it is there, it does not hold up for more than 2-3 minutes. As her desire is more now, I have not been able to satisfy her, leading to psychological problem for both. My questions are :

1. Can I use Viagra or the equivalent to overcome the above problem?

2. Whether the masturbation I once indulged in, has arousal and ejaculation problems.
3. How long normally should the penis inside the vagina last before ejaculation ? Mine is hardly 6-7 oscillations and that it is all over.

Neither of us have any problem with BP, sugar, heart. Even my office/home atmosphere Is very cool, no stress. Despite my "disappointing" performance in bed my wife and I are happy on all other fronts. We are not taking any medication.

Could you please help us.

Here are a few facts that all men over 40 should know

(1) Erection takes longer to occur as you grow older and reqires manual stimulation, preferably by the partner. (2) The erection can at times subside for no particular reason. (3) The semen may not be accompanied by spasmodic ejaculation but trickels out; at times no ejaculation occurs. (4) The quantity (of semen) may be very little: And finally (5) The refractory period (viz. the return of desire) is longer than what it used to be at 20. In your case I would suggest you go to an urologist (or andrologist) who will check your prostate for enlargement. Also have a blood sugar level and urine test (for Infection) done. These may also be the causes behind the premature ejaculation. In reply to your specific queries: (1) you can and it may help but start after consulting a doctor; (2) absolutely not; (3) no fixed time, depends upon the stimuatlion.

Your problems is not because of masturbation. The desired duration of intercourse varies for each couple. In general, it should last as long as is required for the satisfaction of both partners. You can use Viagra in the dose of 50 or 100 mg, 1 hour before intercourse. Additionally, there are several medicines that can be used to delay ejaculation. These can be prescribed for you by an andrologist after evaluation of your problem.

Get Warmth and Love Back in Your Home by Feng-Shui

Fighting all the time? Irritated, grumpy, cursing under your breath? From a Feng Shui perspective, there are some areas in the home that could be turning up the heat, causing conflict between you and your husband. Try to incorporate a cure a day and record your results.

Resolve quarrels and arguments

Examine the bedroom. Is it full of colour or does the room give you a feeling of warmth and comfort? Are the walls painted red or a bright yellow? Were the bedsheets and bed purchased with another lover? Write down all the observations of your bedroom.

- The walls should be painted a nice, soft, romantic colour. Greens and blues are good for the bedroom.
- Replace the bedsheets with new soft linen. Pink and green are great colours to open your hearts for better communication.
- Invest in a new mattress if you did not purchase it as a couple. If finances are an issue, change the mattress to remove old arguments.
- Place your bed against a wall, farthest from the door.

You and your spouse should have a good view of the door.

- Have a sturdy bedframe. No frames that wobble.
- Have a minimum of two pillows on the bed. Pillows should always be in multiples of two.
- Locate the southwest corner in the bedroom. Decorate it to symbolise growth and harmony in your relationship. *Options*: Happy photo of you and your spouse. Objects in pairs - eg two pink candle holders.
- Go to all the southwest corners in the home and see what all lie in corners. Are they vacant or filled with clutter? Clean out all the southwest corners and place a vibrant plant or objects in pairs.
- Organise and clean the front entrance. Have a meandering path to the other areas of the home. If the hallway is filled with chaos and unfinished projects, it will most likely spark friction.
- Organise and clutter free the entire home. Invest in a house that's cleaner, if time is an issue.
- Play soft music or nature sounds. Have a CD player that can continually repeat the music while you are not at home. The sounds will permeate through the house and give you a welcome as you enter.
- Place a few lavender plants in the front entrance. The scent of lavender pomotes peace and calmness.
- The bedroom is the most important room to begin applying the Feng Shui cures. If the home is relaxing and comforting, there will be fewer fights and more discussions of your problems.

Frigidity

'Frigidity' implies sexual unresponsiveness towards sex and, here, either of the partners can be at fault, but a lady partner is often made the scapegoat. Women of frigid nature are called 'cold' women who do not respond to sexual advances of men, and end up as passive non-performers during intercourse. Those who get easily excited and quickly submit to sex are called 'hot' women. Similarly men can also be categorised under the said divisions. Here, the point, under discussion, is sexual unresponsiveness when either of the partners fails to measure up to the sexually heightened, voluptuous sprees and advances of the other partner . The restatement of one-sided sexual excitement is premature ejaculation, thus leaving the other partner mid-way to reel under pangs of instigated sex pleasure.

It is necessary to point out that desire to have sex is a paramount factor and if there is no desire in both the partners, coition is merely a formality or an obligation or compulsion—it is only a meeting of bodies but not of minds. For a successful, and satiating sex, meeting of body and mind is of utmost necessity. Ejaculation is no guarantee for a satisfactory sex nor can it be termed as 'equal indulgence.'

Sex is not intended to be performed in isolation of body and mind. You can satisfy your sex appetite by indulging in other means also, but you won't say 'you have enjoyed it fully'. There is room for partial or casual enjoyment—it is either complete enjoyment or none at all. One-sided sex is a matter of sheer discharging an imposed (social) obligation in respect of your partner or your own self.

There could be following gradational stages of frigidity viz.

1. The woman may show or actually be indifferent toward intercourse (sexual) and may indulge and participate in it simply as a part of her duty towards her husband. In such a situation, she neither abhors nor dislikes option but, all the same, she never enjoys it.
2. The woman does not reach her orgasm, even though she enjoys it. There is a feeling that her participation is quite normal and also that woman's performance is also identical so far as intensity and pleasure are concerned.
3. She may nurture a positive repugnance for sexual intercourse but her body 'freezes' even on an idea of having a coitus. she is merely a passive participant.
4. Fear coitus, especially in young ladies who nurture baseless feelings and suffer from most or any one the following symptomatic factors, viz. :

Any physical problem like headache, pain in breasts and nipples, small breasts, aching in body, palpitation, giddiness, depression, hystereal fits on insertion of male penis, abnormal length and thickness of penis, pain on penile insertion, crying, trembling, nervosity, discharges from vagina, colliquative (debilitating) sweating, etc.

Some women are scared of when a surgeon probes fingers into her vagina. Even the idea of male penerating his penis into her vagina may send shivers down her spine, cause spasms in vagina.

In either case, it is the fear of penetration that triggers frigidity syndrome.

A few ladies remain cool to sexual intercourse because they would hate to bear a child lest their beauty is marred or their figure is spoiled. Such ladies avoid their husbands and pretend one excuse or the other in order to avoid coitus.

This, in fact, is not directly related to any kind Of frigidity but is merely an excuse to abstain from sex. These ladies often complain of pain in body, skin rash, itching of vulva, headache, back pain, etc., so that their husbands may not compel them to have an intercourse. Going to sleep or pretending sleepiness is a common excuse of such reluctant ladies. In fact, such excuses are employed as 'escape routes' to avoide or get rid of coitus.

Frigidity also stems from following contributory factors, apart from the ones already indicated above :-

☞ Inhuman and beastial behaviour of male members with mothers, sisters and also discriminatory treatment.

☞ Organic incompetence.

☞ Inbuilt psycho phobia about intercourse, that it is a filthy, derogatory human instinct that underscores, demeans and degrades a woman's status and that woman is treated merely as a sex-tool.

☞ Lack of proper sex knowledge. She has no idea of male and female sex organs and the individual utility and functions of each organ.

☞ Fear of rupture of hymen or if the same has already been ruptured in premarital period, she is suspicious that her husband may suspect her virginity.

☞ Even ignorance of male, in respect of sexual posture and foreplay, drive a woman away from sexual indulgence. Here, the male member should play his role to introduce variety into coital postures and foreplay.

☞ In crowded families and that too when there is no place for privacy in a joint family, women generally abhor and avoid sex. The problem is more grave in tradition bound families where husband-wife cannot eat together nor go out for a walk nor talk to each other. Such indirectly imposed restrictions inhibit a woman's sexual urges, resulting in her frigidity.

Sterlity and Infertility

Sterility

The term 'sterility' means inability to ave (or conceive) children but applies equally to men also who are unable to impregnate a woman in order to enable to conceive. But the term is applied frequently in case of women only. Sterility may be caused by following factors :

- Removal of ovaries/fallopian tubes.
- Non-production of ovum.
- Sexual unresponsiveness.
- Deranged position of uterus.
- Some ailments of chronic nature.
- Some hormonal disturbances.
- Frequent abortions.
- Consequence of some accident, etc.

Due to advances made in surgical spheres, sterility can be removed and cured if basic cause pertains to some organic defect. In most of the cases, it is the man who is at fault and not the woman. No doubt, atrophy of fallopian tube is still an unresolved problem but other organic defects can be successfully encountered. An adept gynaecologist can easily deduce the cause of sterility and remove the cause by surgical or other means, but timely detection and proper treatment is of paramount importance; hence corrective and curative measures must not be delayed.

Certain ladies nurture innate hatred towards male sex, due to which factor they fail to reach orgasm, thereby impeding the process of onset of pregnancy. Inbuilt inhibitions, fear psychosis, like enormous length of male penis, imagined pain during coitus, resulting in spasms, fits or pains or even avoidance of coitus, are the other factors that could render a woman sterile. The husband should try to set at rest all the fears, inhibitions and imagined problems by sustained persuasion, love, affection, sympathy and reassurance. He should not behave like a stud, but a sympathetic, considerate and caring husband. Rest of the problems can be taken care of by the doctor. If there is a close rapport between both the partners, most of the related problems to sterility can be solved.

Infertility

Here, inability to impregnate is the main cause and in over 90% cases, it is the husband (man) who is at fault. Truly speaking the two terms, viz sterility and infertility in a sense, are two sides of the coins, but cause of malady lies with the husband who has weak sperms which are not potent enough to cause conception. In most of the cases, woman is found to be quite fertile to bear a child by conceiving but is failed, quite often, by her male partner who either does not or cannot reach orgasm or suffers from premature ejaculation in which case the poor lady is left in the lurch. Such a situation causes family problems, feuds between husband and wife, psychic upsets and mental agitation (in women) and a sense of self-condemnation and inferiority (in the males). I have seen myself many family lives shattered due to sexual incompetence of men who either suffer from some psychological complex, sense of shame or have some organic or psychic problem as the underlying causes.

A sensible wife should reassure her husband in this regard and never let him feel demeaned or slighted. She should co-operate with him and help him in maintaining his self-confidence. It is absolutely an imprudent and immature approach to blame each other, instead of having mutual understanding. Healthy looking men are not necessarily potent men. Actually physical appearance and physical structure have nothing to do with virility and sexual performance or competence of a male.

Irrespective of sex, if either of the partners had indulged in self-vice or onanism in adolescence or until they were married or had premarital sexual relations, had been suffering from some venereal disease or indulged in homosexual or heterosexual (free) love, are liable to suffer from syndrome of infertility. All venereal diseases are now fully curable, organic problems can be coached by medicines, operations or psychological treatment.

Sex News

The Good, The Bad & The Sexy

The trouble with most bad porn movies (and magazines) is that they focus on just 2 (okay, sometimes 3) areas of the body. Follow this route and sex can get about as exciting as doing the laundry. To be a better lover, you need more finesse and some knowledge about human anatomy—the libido turning on kind, below, hyped bits and parts, and the 2 (unsung) erotic spots you really should be going for.

What is Hyped : Breasts

Boobies in all shapes and sizes are wondrous things when they're natural. Silicone-filled look good, but can feel more like those red rubber balls from gym class than flesh. Breasts can suffer from PMT tenderness, too.

What's Hot : Thighs

Women hate' em, which is why men should love'em. Lavish them with a little praise and attention. She'll be more comfortable with her body and consider you a God among men.

Thighs also have a practical application. Besides separating knees from her lap, they can be used to improve her sex skills, squeeze them together repeatedly and she'll indirectly strengthen her vaginal muscles making them more powerful during sex (a lazy woman's version of Kegel's exercises). It will also cause a rush of blood to the area, arousing her on the spot.

What's Hyped : Penis

Granted that a man loves having his penis touched, but there can be times when you can touch too much, so that he comes too soon.

What's Hot : His perineum

What's that ? The ridge between the back of the scrotum and the anus. Light caresses with the fingers or the tongue can drive a man wild. Because the nerves in the perineum are part of the sexual nervous system, pressure with the fingers tips at the mid point of the ridge, can often induce, or restore a flagging erection.

Talking Sex

Want to set the bed on fire tonight ? Start your "lovemaking" early in the evening. Go to dinner at a fancy restaurent. "During the meal, you're allowed to talk only about sexual fantasies," suggests Patricia Love, Ed.D., author of Hot Monogamy. "There's something very erotic about being public and being surreptitious about your seuxality." Bonus mission: Order foods that are delicious and lascivious at the same time—eg. delicately cooked fish, stewed ripe fruit, icecream, chocolate.

JUST MAKE OUT : Another libido firer : Have a make-out date in a car at least an hour long, with no below-the-belt contact. It's a fun. teenage-style !

Flirting

"Flirting is acting amorously without serious intent," says Susan Rabin, author of *How to Attract Anyone Anytime, Anyplace*.

Rabin, a therapist and communcations coach, has been teaching the art of flirting since 1984. Most people come to her because they're shy. They want to level the playing field, to learn the same social skills that other come by naturally.

"The difference between a shy person and a flirt," Rabin explains, "is that a shy person is thinking about himself or herself, while a flirt is thinking about otners." Ask questions, and people will be attracted by you, she says. "Don't tune in to WIIFM : What's in it for Me ?"

Another trick - SOFTEN : Smile, Open posture, Forward lean, Touch, Eye contact, and Nod.

Rabin's most important lesson : "Consider rejection a favour." With each one your'll learn to eliminate boo-boos and become more adept at social interactions.

Painful Breasts ?

Breast pain is common—and usually nothing to fear. Unless you're pregnant, the usual cause of breast pain (mastalgia) is fibrocystic changes in the breast. These are physical changes in the structure of the breast tissue that are typically caused by premenstrual hormonal changes.

Breast pain is also extremely coomon in women in their thirties and forties. At this age, women enter premenopause, the decade before menopause. During this time, hormonal levels undergo increased fluctuation.

Other culprits are oral contraceptives and caffeine. Cut back on coffee and try taking extra vitamin B. But if symptoms persist see your doctor.

Like Father, Like Husband

It's often said that women tend to marry men who resemble dear old Dad. Now comes a study to support that belief. Volunteers were asked to pick out family members within sets of unlabeled photos. By seeking out similar faces, participants were able to match wives with their spouses

31 per cent of the time and husbands with their fathers-in-law almost 40 per cent of the time. The percentage of correct matches for both sets of pictures was much higher than would be expected by chance. What's more, the photographed wives had - so the image been adopted matchers weren't using inherited resemblances to an advantage. Why might women seek a second father figure? Study co author Glenn Weisfeld, Ph.D., a psychologist at Wayne State University, says a learning process called imprinting may bum a copy of "Dad as ideal man" into daughters' young brains. Imprinting could nudge them toward mates who look familiar—that is, like family and therefore may share genetic traits with them. That may have an upside: Couples with similar genes seem to have slightly lower miscarriage rates, he says. Of course, though, there is such a thing as too much similarity. Marriage between very close relatives brings risk, such as an increased chance of disability in offspring. "But once you get to the level of first or second cousin, the risk seems to dissipate," Weisfeld says." And there may even be benefits."

Power Booster Nutrients for Men

Men need more of just about every essential nutrient than women. Here are the nine most important vitamins and minerals that every man should know about.

Which vitamins do you need most, and how much do you need ? *Men's Health* went to the experts for the answers. But first, an interesting footnote : Men and women have differing nutritional needs. In fact, the U.S. Food and Drug Administration puts out separate men's and women's lists of Recommended Dietary Allowances (RDA) for vitamins and minerals. And men need more of just about every essential nutrient that women do. Why ? Quite simply, because we're bigger. We have more muscle and burn more calories than women do. And those of us who are fit and active, in particular, need higher quantities of certain key nutrients.

Further, getting enough of the right vitamins, minerals can helps fight problems we men are at especially high risk for, such as elevated cholesterol, hypertension, coronary heart disease, stroke, certain cancers and kidney stones.

Here, in alphabetical order, are the nine nutrients men need most.

Chromium

This vital mineral can cut cholesterol, boost endurance in athletes and help body-builders gain muscle and lose fat. The average man needs at least 50 micrograms, of chromium a day, but active men should get 100 to 200 micrograms, according to Richard Anderson, Ph.D., of the U.S. Department of Agriculture Human Nutrition Research Centre. "You'll have a hard time getting this much from foods," he says. Your best source is a multivitamin / mineral complex that includes chromium. Next best is one or two chromium-fortified tablets of brewer's yeast daily.

Fiber

Technically, fiber's not a nutrient, since it passes through the body undigested. But eating fiber substantially reduces cholesterol and may help lower blood pressure. A high-fiber diet may lower your risk of colon cancer (the third most common kind for men) and can control sugar levels in diabetics. Fiber may even help you lose weight by filling you up without a lot of calories. Two medium-sized apples will give you 14 of the recommended 18 to 35 daily grams of dietary fiber you need. You also get fiber from whole-grain breads and breakfast cereals; brown rice, strawberries, pears and vegetables, especially ones with edible stalks and stems such as broccoli and carrots.

Magnesium

This mineral plays a key role in regulating the heart-beat—studies show that getting enough may protect men against heart disease as well as bring down high blood pressure. Magnesium also boosts fertility by making sperm more vigorous. You'll get about two-thirds of your daily requirement of magnesium from a breakfast of two cups of shredded wheat, skim milk and a banana. Baked potatoes, beans, nuts, oatmeal, peanut butter, whole-wheat spaghetti, leafy vegetables and seafood are also magnesium rich.

Vitamin A

Studies find vitamin A can have significant immunity-boosting and anticancer effects. And, yes, just as your mother told you, it helps maintain good vision. A ½-cup serving of steamed carrots supplies almost four times a man's daily recommended intake of 1,000 milligrams. Other good sources are liver, dairy products, fish, tomatoes, apricots, etc. Vitamin A is easy to get from your diet and extremely toxic in high doses, so experts recommend avoiding supplements

Vitamin B_6

This necessary nutrient is a powerful immune booster, and some studies suggest it may prevent skin and bladder cancer. Additionally, B_6 protects against the formation of kidney stones (a problem that afflicts twice as may men as women) and can help prevent restless sleep. You need only two milligrams of vitamin B_6 daily—about the amount in two large bananas. Active men need a few milligrams more, since it's burned up during exercise, says Paul Tremble, Ph.D., assistant professor of nutritional biochemistry at Purdue University. Other dietary sources include chicken and fish, liver, potatoes, avocados and sunflower seeds. High does of B_6 supplements can be toxic over time, so experts recommend taking not more than 50 milligrams a day.

Vitamin c

It boosts immunity; may help prevent cancer, heart disease and stroke; promotes healthy gums and teeth; prevents cataracts; hastens wound healing; counteracts asthma; and may help overcome infertility in men. Keeping your body well supplied with vitamin C may also slow the aging process.

Brocoli, cantaloupe, green peppers and grapefruit juice are good dietary sources, but supplements won't harm you, as this vitamin's not toxic in high does. Researcher Earl Dawson, Ph.D., of the University of Texas Medical Branch, says 200 to 300 milligrams a day should be adequate. Many researchers think you'll short-change yourself on vitamin C with the RDA of 60 milligrams (the amount in ½ cup of fresh orange juice), particularly when it comes to warding off the common cold, the most well known of C's benefits.

If you smoke, you probably need extra vitamin C. Smokers have lower levels of the vitamin in their blood. No one knows why, but the implication is that their bodies need more C and thus are using more.

Vitamin e

Studies show vitamin E lowers cholesterol, prevents buildup of artery-clogging plaque, boosts immunity, cleanses the body of pollutants and prevents cataracts. There's lots of vitamin E in almonds, peanuts and pecans, but it's hard to get enough of this nutrient from your diet. Fortunately, supplements are safe in doses much higher than the 10-milligram RDA. Biochemist Max Horwitt, Ph.D., of the St. Louis University School of Medicine, takes 269 milligrams daily and considers the amount safe.

Water

It's the most essential of all nutrients, especially if you're muscular: Muscle contains almost three times more water than fat. (The average man's body is 40 percent muscle, while the average woman's is 23 percent). Water lubricants joints, regulates temperature and provides the body with minerals and essential fluids. The average man should get at least two quarts a day, or about eight glasses, "If you're physically active, you could easily need to double that," says Georgia Kostas, a registered dietitian and doctor of nutrition at the

Cooper Clinic. You also get water from food : Bread is about 36 percent water, a potato, 80 percent.

Zinc

Getting enough zinc ensures that your sex drive, potency and fertility stay in shape. Zinc's been used experimentally to treat impotence, and it has a profound influence on the body's ability to heal wounds and resist disease. Men tend to get only about two-thirds the RDA of 15 milligrams, particularly if we're active. That's because when men sweat, we lose more since than women. One four-ounce helping of lean beef provides almost half the daily zinc needs. Other good sources are turkey, seafood, cereals and beans. Too much zinc can hinder the work of other minerals, so experts recommend taking no more than one 15-milligram supplement a day.

Get more fiber

Insoluble or soluble ? It doesn't matter how you get your fiber. What's important is that you do get it. "People eat so little fiber, we'll take anything, "says Dr. Blackburn. "Whatever you can find—some peas in your stew—put them in!"

A high-fiber diet fills you up without filling you out, keeps you regular, helps lower your cholesterol level and may help reduce the risk of colon cancer. The nutritionists advocate getting at least 20 grams per day. A breakfast of oatmeal, whole-wheat toast, a pear and a banana would give you more than half that amount. The highest-fiber foods are fruits, vegetables, whole grains and legumes.

Fiber Champs

These ten foods are loaded with fiber.

1. All Bran with Extra Fiber, ½ cup : 13.8 gms.

2. Kidney beans, cooked, ½ cup : 6.9 gms.
3. Wheat "lite" bread, 2 slices : 5.6 grams.
4. Turnips, cooked, ½ cup : 4.8 grams.
5. Green peas, frozen, cooked, ½ cup : 4.3 gms.
6. Pears, canned, ½ cup : 3.7 grams.
7. Raspberries, fresh, 1 cup : 3.3 grams.
8. French-style green beans, cooked, ½ cup : 2.8 grams.
9. Granny Smith apple, 1 small : 2.8 grams.
10. Popcorn, 3 cups: 2.0 grams.

High Calcium Cocktails

You can reduce high blood pressure by eating more low-fat dairy products and drinking lots of fortified orange juice, suggest studies out of Arizona State University. Men who ate a high-calcium diet (600 milligrams more than the Recommended Dietary Allowance) for six weeks saw their high blood pressure readings drop dramatically.

Salt

Your body needs a mere 500 milligrams of salt - 1/16 teaspoon - per day. You can get that in a cup of instant soup or a few handfuls of honey-roasted peanuts. The average American man eats 20 times that amount. When you begin to approach 20 to 30 grams per day (which, incidentally, is what the average Japanese consumes), you get to a level that may put you at risk for high blood pressure, arterial damage and even stroke.

Commonest Rules of Diet

1. Avoid excess salts and sugar.
2. Keep low the consumption of red meat, primarily beef and lamb and substitute fish and poultry, legumes and grains, nuts and seeds.
3. Substitute low-fat milk for whole milk, low-fat cheese

for high-fat cheese.

4. Substitute polyunsaturated margarine and vegetable oils for utter, lard and bacon fat.
5. Eat plenty of fruits, and green leafy, as well as yellow vegetables, raw and cooked.

General Health

1. Get seven or eight hours' sleep at night.
2. Eat breakfast—especially high fibre foods and fruits.
3. Keep weight normal in relation to height.
4. Avoid smoking.
5. Exercise regularly.
6. Drink only in moderation (a glass or two of wine or beer per day and spirits only occassionally).
7. Burn the candle at only one end (i.e., if you work too hard, then don't play too hard, or if you play too hard, then don't work too hard; alternate periods of overexertion with periods of rest, and periods of laziness with periods of self-galvanishing).

Attitude Towards Self-Love, Confidence and Body Language

Self - Love

Some people think it's a sin to love yourself. They consider those who love themselves to be selfish, conceited and rather unpleasent. But they're mistaken. They confuse self-love with false pride and narcissism (being in love with yourself) which is quite a different matter. Vanity and arrogance are usually a form of bravado engaged in by people who love themselves too little and are trying to cover it up.

If you don't love yourself you'll have no sense of self-worth, and no feeling of acceptenace or belonging.

Furthermore, your capacity for loving others is directly related to how much love you have for yourself. You can't share anything you don't have. How can you truly love another if you don't feel worthy of giving and receving love ? Impossible.

The belief that you need to be different from how you are in order to be loved causes a great deal of misery. Unless you are happy within, you'll never be truly satisfied with what you do. Loving yourself unconditionally is the key to happiness. But you don't have to be perfect : the most loved person in the world makes mistakes ! You don't even have to do your best. You don't have to prove anything. You're all right because yo're all right, and lovable exactly as you are.

'It's a funny thing about life : if you refuse to accept anything less than the best, you very often get it.—W. Somerset Maugham

Reflect on your attitude to loving yourself. It is OK to love yourself ? Or do you consider it sinful ? Arrogant, conceited ? If so, from where does this attitude come ?

Write down this sentence :

'If only I were....... then I'd be lovable.'

Quickly, without thinking about it too hard, fill in the gap with whatever comes to mind. Examine what you've written. Does it really make sense ?

Think of someone or several people you know who are loud, boastful, arrogant and vain. In your opinion do these people truly love themselves ? Or are they in love with themselves ? Is their outward display nothing more than a cover up ?

Regularly pamper yourself. Treat yourself to an occassional massage, aromatherapy, sauna, a long soak in the bath, reflexology, a manicure, whatever you fancy. Not only does it help recharge your batteries, but it also reminds you that you deserve the very best.

Relax your body. Calm your mind. Imagine there is someone there with you, who loves you, really loves you. This could be a living or deceased persona, a spiritual being whom you admire, such as Krishna, Jesus, Buddha or Mohammed, or a guardian angel. Welcome them. 'Feel' their presence.

Now imagine that this person is telling you how much he or she loves you and all the good things they see in you. Listen carefully. How do you feel ?

When you return to full altertness, describe the experience in your notebook.

Use these affirmations :

'I am worthy of all the good in my life.'

'I am open and accepting of myself and others.'

'I am loving, lovable and loved.'

'I feel warm and loving towards myself at all times.'

Practise TFM - Time for Me. Make time for yourself every day, for relaxing, doing as your please, having fun. This sends a powerful message to the subconscious that you deserve it and you're worth it. Besides if you don't make time for yourself, who else is going to make time for you?

When you learn to love yourself, change always takes palce. Not always immediately—but it will.

Confidence-building activities

The following activities are terrific confidence boosters. Obviously some will appeal to you more than others. For instance, if you enjoy dancing and you'r good at it, you'll probably feel that taking dancing lessons is unnecessary. But if you hate dancing, lack confidence on the dance floor and find it difficult to express yourself physically, the very idea may traumatise you.

Why do most of us find it hard to put ourselves on the line ? Usually because we're frigthtened of showing ourselves up. But with high self-esteem we don't worry about making fools of ourselves in front of others because we know instinctively that this is not a disaster.

So what if you don't succed first time ? The obstacles don't grow any bigger but you do ! With a positive self-image you can fail completely and still feel good about yourself.

- Because I'm OK I can make mistake. I can fail and still feel good about myself.
- I am enthusiastic about life and filled with energy and purpose.

'Failure is the opportunity to begin again, more intelligently.'

—Henry Ford

Join a speakers' club or enroll on a public speaking course. Speaking to an audience is many people's number one fear, but even if you never intend giving a speech, attending speaking classes will do wonders for your confidence.

Take singing lessons. Join a choir or small singing group and sing in public. Better still, do is solo. Alternatively, join a drama group.

Take dancing lessons—disco, rock 'n' roll, ballroom, it doesn't matter. Use your body. Become more physically expressive. Bear in mind you're not doing it to impress, but to feel more at ease with the way you move. Playing chess / cards with family and friends, or better still, strangers, can bring the same rewards.

Take a self-defence course. You get a wonderful feeling of confidence from knowing that you could deal with a physical attack if necessary.

If you're shy, join a club or society that brings you into contact with others. Choose one that enables you to pursue your favourite hobby or something at which you excel. We all need contact with other poeple and, no matter how shy you are, you won't cure it by hiding away.

Do a bungee jump or go skydiving. Take up rock climbing, hang gliding or white water rafting. Challenging yourself physically is a wonderful way of building confidence.

Every evening allow ten mintues to reflect on the day's events. Note the positive aspects of the day. Dwell on the most enjoyable moments as if savouring a delicious morsel of food.

Saturday night failure

Richard was thoroughly miserable. At 35 this successful entrepreneur was still single and lonely. 'I work late most eveing,' he said, 'because I dread going home. There's nothing to go home to.' He had never had a girlfrind, his only sexual contacts being with prostitutes, for which he felt dirty and ashamed.

He believed one of his main problems lay in his inabillity to join in the dancing at discos and nightclubs. He had been to many down the years, but try as he might stepping onto the dance floor, he would stand at the bar watching people dancing and later leaving together, if he stayed that long. Usually he sloped off well before closing time.

Richard was encouraged to enrol for dancing lessons, and taught how to use anchoring. In stages he visualised himself arriving at the nightclub, chatting to people and buying drinks, using the 'cool, calm and confident' trigger if he felt his anxiety levels rising. Then he visualised himself, calmly stepping twords the dance floor and moving easily - nothing too flamboyant at first - then appraoching an attractive woman and dancing with her.

Then he took the plunge. At first he was terrified, but within a few weeks he was able to do everything for which he had set out.

CONFIDENT BODY LANGUAGE

When you move confidently and carry your body confidently, you not only feel more confident but others assume that you are.

You may be surprised to learn that only 7 % of the information you transmit to others is in the language you use. The remainder comes from :

- 38% How you speak—quality of voice, accent, voice projection, emphasis, epxression, pace, volume, pitch etc.
- 55% Body language—posture, position, eye contact, facial expression, head and body movements, gestures, touch, etc.

Whereas people often try to disguise their true feelings in their utterances, they communicate them freely through their non-verbals. When your body language tells a different story from your spoken words, guess which is believed ? The answer is, your body language. **It imparts eight times as much information.**

Pay more attention to how you use your body. Poor movement and posture restricts breathing, tightens the muscles and brings about skeletal disorders.

One of the best ways of improving your posture is to practise the Alexander Technique, a wonderful method for detecting and releasing muscular tension. It involves moving with the back straight, gaze gently fixed straight ahead, shoulders back but releaxed, ears, shoulders, hips and ankles in line. This has the effect of lengthening and widening the spine, giving the lungs a chance to work better. This is the epitome of a confident posture. Moreover, regular practitioners also find themselves mentally calmer and more confident than before.

'No one has even seen a cock crow with its head down.'

Alonzo Newton Benn

Stand in front of a mirror. Hold your head up, back straight, shoulders back, looking straight ahead. Try to make yourself look bigger, as if you're taking up more space—good posture automatically takes up more space. Now walk briskly and confidently around the room. How do you feel ?

A proud, upright stance makes you look more important, even if you're not especially tall. It makes you look younger and slimmer too.

Now do the opposite. Droop your shoulders, head down, looking at the floor. Make yourself smaller, as if your body is closing in on itself. How confident do you feel now ?

Hand and arm movements are very expressive. Learn to use your hands for emphasis, and keep hand movements smooth and flowing. Avoid :

- Folding your arms or wrapping them around yourself (like a cuddle). This indicates a closed, defensive attitude and makes you appear unappraochable.
- Placing your hands in your pockets.
- Tapping on surfaces such as tables and desks with your fingers or on the back of your other hand.
- Fidgeting, scratching, wringing your hands (which shows tension).
- Touching your face or neck. This reveals discomfort

or embarrassment.

Become aware of all your mannerisms and gestures. If possible video yourself, watch carefully and make adjustments.

Eyes are very expressive

- Lively, sparkling eyes are attractive. They say, 'Talk to me, I'm appraochable.
- Looking away shows disinterest or deviousness.
- Looking down conveys submission.

Confident people make more frequent eye contact than people who are unsure of themselvs, so develop a steady gaze. When you enter a room move arond comfortably, smile and make gentle eye contact with everyone; not too much, not too little.

Your breathing is very important. You can calm down instantly and become less tense and anxious by taking your attention to the breath, slowing and depending it.

Practise calming the breath. Slow breaths and a steady gaze, confined with an anchor such as 'Cool, calm and relaxed', can combat nervosness any time, whereever you are and whoever you'r with.

Make better use of your personal space. Try to make yourself bigger. The more room you appear to occupy, the more confident and important you appear. But moving too close to others is unsettling, so don't get too near.

To 'steepling'. Join your fingertips to form what looks like a church steeple. This communicates authority and gives the imprssion you're sure of what you're saying.

Controlling Mind

Mind control means the learning of methods of influcening the subconscious mind. For this, you need to have some knowledge of how the inner mind works and of its working-up. Ending its activitites that may be affecting you adversely and putting it to work for your with all of its great powes can make a great change in your life.

Mind control enables you to make many chnages in yourself, which will be of the utmost benefit to you. This means the learning of ways to influence your inner mind.

Holding a soft pencil or a ball-point pen in your hand, the inner mind can take control of the muscles of your hand and can write intelligibly without your being aware of what it is writing. You can be reading a book while you had writes. A few very good "automators" have been able to read with the conscious mind while the right hand writes about something, and at the same time the left hand writes on some other subject. Thus, three different mental activities can be carried on at the same time ! The operation of a Ouija board is just a variation of automatic writing. Those who believe in spiritualism think that the hand is controlled by some spirit and that through the Ouija board information can be gained from the spirit world. More probably, it is knowlege or fantasy coming from the subconscious.

The Value of a Smile

It costs nothing, but creates much.

It enriches those who receive, without impoverishing those who give.

It happens in a flash and the memory of it sometimes lasts forever.

None are so rich they can get along without it, and none so poor but are richer for its benefits.

It creates happiness in the home, fosters goodwill in a business, and is the countersign of friends.

It is rest to the waerily, daylight to the discouraged, sunshine to the sad, and nature's best antidote for trouble.

Yet it cannot be bought, begged, borrowed, or stole, for it is something that is no earthly good to anybody till it is given away.

And if in the last-minute rush of Christmas buying some of our salespeople should be too tired to give you a smile, may we ask you to leave one of yours ?

For nobody needs a smile so much as those who have none left to give !

Six Ways to Make People Like You

PRINCIPLE 1

Become genuinely interested in other people.

PRINCIPLE 2

Smile

PRINCIPLE 3

Remember that a person's name is to that person the sweetest and most imporant sound in any language.

PRINCIPLE 4

Be a good lisener. Enocourage others to talk about themselves.

PRINCIPLE 5

Talk in terms of the other person's interests.

PRINCIPLE 6

Make the other person feel important—and do it sincerely.

Queries for the Married Life

The following questionnaire is based on Gottman's seven principles of making marriage work. Answer true or false for each, then score yourself at the conclusion. If you're feeling brave, have your partner take the same test and see how your compare.

1. I can list my partner's major aspiration and hopes in life. T F
2. I know my partner's current major worries. T F
3. I know the three most special times in my spouse's life. T F
4. I can easily list the three things I most admire about my partner. T F
5. I often touch or kiss my spouse affectionately. T F
6. Our sex life is generally satisfying. T F
7. I look forward to spending my free time with my partner. T F
8. My partner is one of my best friend. T F
9. My partner tells me when he or she has had a bad day. T F
10. I am genuinely interested in my spouse's opinion. T F
11. I usually learn a lot from my spouse even when we disagree. T F
12. I feel I have an important say when we make decisions. T F

13. I can admit that I am wrong. T F
14. Even when we disagree, we can maintain a sense of humour. T F
15. My spouse is good at soothing me when I get upset. T F
16. My partner and I are a good team. T F
17. When we argue, winning isn't my objective. T F
18. I accept that there are issues we will never resolve. T F
19. We share many similar values in our roles as husband and wife. T F
20. We share many happy memories. T F

Scoring : 13 or more true answers : You have a solid relationship that will probably endure until both of your are toothless and incontinent. Fortunately, you'll still be so in love that neither of you will notice.

7 to 12 true answers : This is a pivotal time in your relationship. There are many strengths you can build upon, but there are also some weaknesses that need tending. It's time to put down that TV remote and get away for the weekend.

6 or fewer true answers: You may be in danger of breaking apart. If this scares you, you probably still value the relationship enough to try to save it. Honest talk is needed. But if that's not possible, you may want to consult a therapist or marriage counsellor.

Marital Red Alerts

"Every marriage ought to be equipped with a built-in early-warning system," Says Gottman. "This allows you to talk about issues while they're still minor." The following marital red alert detector will help you to do just that. More than two "yes" answers means trouble is brewing, and you should talk about it now.

1. When I'm with my partner, I often want to be

somewhere else.

2. There is tension between us.
3. My partner has little idea what I'm thinking.
4. I wish we were closer right now.
5. My partner has wanted to be alone a lot lately.
6. We've been fighting more often.
7. There hasn't been much fun or joy in our lives lately.
8. Small issues have a tendency to escalate.
9. We have been hurting each other's feelings.
10. We really need to talk.

Courtesy - H & N

Post Coital Pleasure

Having sex puts men to sleep but wakes women up. Why, you wonder? Unfortunately, the cocktail of sex hormones released after both women and men climax can have totally opposite effects on our post sex wish list. "Studies show that following intercourse, the male brain often goes into a rest state—he feels drained and tired—while the woman's brain is stimulated and desires bonding," explains Michael Gurian, therapist and author of *What Could He Be Thinking: How A Man's Mind Really Works*.

Fear not, though. We've overcome those biological obstacles and identified after-play pleasures that will satisfy you both. Some are designed to short-circuit his snooze reflex and electrify his body; others indulge his just-shagged daze while feeding your need for intimacy. Read on to discover the randy moves that will create the most pleasurable and satisfying after-sex moments you have had with your man yet.

Pay him a carnal compliment

Guys are suckers for hearing about their sizzling sex skills. When you mention the mattress moves that drove you wild, it strokes his ego and makes him feel virile. "Men can feel anxious about their performance, so they really want to hear it from you that you had a good time in bed," says

Judy Kuriansky, Ph.D., author of *The Complete Idiot's Guide To A Healthy Relationship*. Your flattering feedback will keep him from dozing he is definitely gonna stay awake for this performance assessment—and help kick-start light conversation, which you may be in the mood for right about now. So recall the evening's erotic events in detail, but don't go too over the top with your carnal confessions. Whenever a girl raves about the sex but doesn't give specifics, I feel like she's blowing smoke up my ass," admits Ewan, 27. To start, you can describe your favourite body lock: "That position where I got on top of you and we both straightened our legs ... WOW!" Or, opt for a little technique approval: "I really liked the way you kept so still while I was climaxing.,,

Your dirty talk will stay with him long after your lacy throng has been retrieved from the ceiling fan. "It leaves a very sexy impression," assures josh, 25. Plus, there is a long-term benefit to this booty wrap-up: it imprints your "Yes, please!" moments in his memory for next time.

Give him a massage

Just because the sex is over doesn't mean it's hands-off. Massage is a great way to maintain that physical connection for you, while prolonging his bliss buzz. Obviously, foreplay hot spots—such as his privates—will be a tender no-go zone. "There's nothing worse than a girl who keeps handling your goods after sex," complains Matt, 27. "It's never a good idea." Remember, you need to unlock the erogenous zones that will keep your guy in a state of ongoing pleasure, not pain.

If you crave a more relaxing and sensual session, position yourself so that you're lying on your side, facing him. "Trace light circles on his torso. Starting at the chest, move around the navel, skim the pelvic bone, and continue back up," says Steve Capellini, massage therapist and author of *Massage For Dummies*. "Or stroke your fingertips from his collarbone down over his chest to his hip bones and back again." These moves allow you to tickle his fancy while still maintaining an intimate post-passion gaze.

When you want him to reciprocate, try to tempt him with a more invigorating touch. Capellini suggests a technique called percussion. Have your guy lie on his stomach and straddle him. "Bounce the sides of your hands or push and tap your fingertips along his back and buttocks," says Capellini. While you enjoy the tactile thrill of having your legs wrapped around him, your touch encourages increased blood flow, making him feel energised rather than drained ... and may even inspire him to return the favour.

Take a shower

When Cosmo asked guys about the most sexalicious thing women could do after getting busy, this was their number-one plea: suggest a shower for two. It's a no brainier. Any situation that has you hot, wet, nude, and invading his personal space is bound to overpower his post coital crash response. "I love being pulled into the shower by my girlfriend after sex. Her wet body rubbing against me its all good,".

Start by taking turns slowly scrubbing each other's back, shoulders and neck. Then press up against your lover for some sexy snuggling under the shower stream, running your slippery, sudsy hands over his back and butt.

The heat-soaked environment not only keeps your bods super-close, but it also actually prolongs the post-orgasmic flush of your just-finished booty session. Here's how: "As the hot water hits your skin, it stimulates blood flow and circulation, which keeps your body feeling aroused," says Sandor Gardos, Ph.D., sexologist based in San Francisco, US.

If all this post-coital closeness inspires something frisky to unfold between you and him, go right there. But ultimately, being so together after being so intimate is often enough of a rush.

Touch Yourself

If the first romp has left you yearning for a repeat performance—but he's totally wiped out—try and turn your attention downstairs for some self-stimulation, and leave the invitation open for him to take over. "Guys need time to recover before they can go again, and this is only made more difficult if they feel pressured," says Kuriansky" So let him know you had an amazing time and that you just want him to be there while you make the most of how aroused you feel."

Whether he joins in or not, guys love to watch, so it's a win-win situation. "A woman touching herself next to me in bed ? That's about as good as life gets," says Christian. Even if your menage-a-moi doesn't tempt him out of retirement, you finish on a high note and he gets a private peep show.

Snuggle up

The ultimate compromise between his and her post-coital carvings is the snuggle up. Being held after sex feels so good for you, while he gets to kick back and indulge his snooze reflex. And the good news is, it's somewhat of a mattress myth that men are turned off by a little after-sex cuddling. "There is an assumption that men are more emotionally detached from intercourse than women are. But a lot of them do want to feel that closeness too," explains Carolynn Hillman, sex therapist based in New York City. Chander, totally agrees lying in bed together and holding my girlfriend after sex is a big part of the buzz."

Of course, if your man isn't a throw his-arms-around-you kind of guy, saying "hold me" sounds kind of lame. Instead, let him settle into a comfortable snoozing position and then wrap his arm around you or spoon him and enjoy that just shagged feeling.

MORE FLIRTING

You can never be too familiar to first, so rediscover your man's playful, sexy side with these tempting triggers.

It's a Two-Way Street

"Women are used to guys making all the moves in the beginning," says Gail E. Wyatt, Ph.D., sex therapist. But once you're together, guys can get lazy. So, tickle his tender spots to provoke a fun rumble or shoot him a coy look from across the bar.

Sex-Up the Boring Stuff

You can turn normally mundane moments into racy exchanges. "Next time you're running errants, steel a well-concealed caress," says Sandra Anne Taylor, author of *Secrets of Attraction*. Or, at the store, say something like, "Want to lick this off me later ?" Chocolate syrup can be so saucy !

Plan a Mystery Date

"Nothing ignites a man's interest faster than intrigue," says Taylor. Give him a time — "See you at eight, Sexy" — but skip the details. His anticipation combines with your sinful grin and subtle body contact will flick the switch on his inner flirt.

Blow His Mind Tip

The second easiest thing to arouse in a man is his spirit of competition. So go ahead, pose him a challenge where you both win. Ask him to guess what kind of lingerie you're wearing, your favourite mattress move, or which of your hands contains a naughty surprise. If he's totally clueless, set a pervy punishment, such as 10 push-ups (naked). Next up, it's his turn to give you a tawdry task.

Food to Enhance Sexual Potency

Food preference is a matter of personal choice, and preference for a particular system of medicine is a matter of faith and conviction which depend largely on your experience. Hereunder, we mention some of the recipes which can keep you sexually active and potent. One may prefer to call such recipes and prescriptions as aphrosdisiacs but they certainly don't belong to the latter category. It is not necessary all persons can derive equal benefits due to the reason that susceptibility, reaction or adverse effects cannot be denied. Hence, be cautious. Better consult some doctor, Vaidya, Hakeem before you embark upon using some formula.

Premature Ejaculation and Impotency

Slice garlic cloves (1/4 kg.) and boil in 2 kgs of milk. When the milk has condensed and bears a semi-liquid (or paste) from, roast the whole content in 250 gms of pure desi ghee (clarified butter oil). Now grind the roasted contents to pulp form, spread on a stainless steel plate, adding some honey to it, and cut into small pieces. Those who get hypersexual, even on thought of having sex, or those who ejaculate even before their penis touches even the outer skirts of vagina, should take about 25-50 gms with hot milk: It will also thicken the semen and won't let is dribble away in a hush. Those who develop some reaction or are prone to garlic reaction should desist from using this recipe. Instead ' such persons should try the following preparation.

Emblical Myrobalan (AMLA)

Take fresh fruit ' remove the stone, and then dry the amla cloves under shade, taking care that it remains free from dust, sun, insects and other impurities. When fully dry, reduce the cloves to a powder form. Now extract juice of fresh amla, in which the amla powder should be immersed, and allowed to dry, as stated above. Fresh amla juice should be ' added seven times (when the powder and juice get fully dried up, then pour juice into it). After the seventh treatment, powder the content to fine pulverised form. and bottle up in a glass bottle. Normal dose is 10 gms thrice daily. While using the powder add 10 gms of *desi ghee* and 5 gms of pure honey. It will thicken semen, raise up your sexual potency, do away with early ejaculation. If after a quick seminal discharge, during first coitus, you take the above dose with hot milk (in-between the relapsing time between two intercourses), you will derive exceptionally more, delayed and satiated enjoyment. It will also improve general health of the body. If ladies use this compound, they will get carried away more to sex and enjoy themselves and also let their husbands also enjoy deeper sex. Already sexually strong and active ladies should avoid using it; as they can cause their mates to ejaculate far earlier than they used to be formerly.

Isabgole

It is available in two form—in the husk form which is white, and the whole form which is blackish—brown. Take whole Isabgole and divest it of all the foreign matters. Now, take a glassful of hot milk and mix about 10 - 15 gms into (2 to 3 teaspoonfuls) in the milk, but don't let the isabgole form into small balls, rather shake it well in the milk. When it has got fully mixed up with milk, it should be sipped, and not gulped. It is claimed that, if a person takes this mixture daily (at night), his semen will thicken, sperms will multiply in count, orgasm will prolong and problem of quick/ premature ejaculation would disappear, but the experiment should be continued for at least 40 days or so.

Date(s)

It is a famous fruit, growing on coastal lands. It has high percentage of sugar; hence diabetics shouldn't use it, when dates are dried, they are called 'Chhoaras'. Boil 4-6 dates (fresh or dried) in milk and when they soften, eat them and drink the milk also. It is a very powerful drink which, if used during winter season, will prove to be an aphrodisiac of high value, as it enhances sexual power and arouses sensuality. It is useful for ladies also—at least to ward off cold and subside ill-effects thereof. Persons of bilious temperament and diabetics should use dates only after seeking medical advice. Even otherwise, fresh dates can be used without milk, or dried dates sliced into small pieces and sucked. Fresh, ripe dates should be fully cleaned, as dust and others particles easily adhere to them. Further, dates with milk can be taken in the morning before and/or after coitus. If taken before coitus it will provide impetus to sex power, if taken after coitus, it will make up for the loses or remove.any sense of weakness felt after ejaculation. If taken in the morning, it will store plenty of energy in the body to enjoy sex. So, in whichever form or at whichever time it is taken, it will always exert salutary effect on you.

Asparagus (Shatavar or Shatavari)

Asparagus should be pounded and reduced to a fine powder. Taken one teaspoonful with hot milk, at least 2 hours prior to anticipated time of sex. It will cause imense erection to penis, impart strength to penis, delay ejaculation, enhance sexual pleasure. It should be used with caution, as it is capable to excite libido to extreme heights and, if taken during daytime, priapism (penile erection) often results.

Black Gram (Kala Chana) & Munakka (Raisins)

Take equal quantity of roasted black grains, adding equal quantity of dried grapes (Munakka, after removing the seeds) and almonds. Take 2 tablespoonfuls daily with hot milk to control early ejaculation, lack of sex power, or power to hold on for longer duration. It imparts virility, removes impotence. It is both a tonic, food and aphrodisiac, but has to be taken daily. Diabetics should reduce quantity of Munakka.

Egg, Honey & Brandy

Beat an egg and vigorously shake the contents. Now mix two teaspoons of honey and a teaspoon of doctor's brandy. It can give you an immediate fillip to your sex power and capacity, cause instant erection, enhance your joy of coital sex (but you should control your sexy lust and desire to full benefit). Certain persons are allergic to use of eggs or even brandy, hence they shouldn't venture to have a try on this prescription.

Alum (Phitkari)

Mix 6 gms of ground alum and 6 gms of borax (suhaga) to 30 - 3 5 drops of Aqua Rose (Gulab Jal). Now, the said mixture is to be boiled in water, making sure that not even a drop falls into it. When entire mixture melts completely, it should be allowed to cool down. (You can use a tight container in the water, fully closed tightly with a lid, to rule out any possibility of entry of water in the mixture). The viscous fluid, so obtained, should be gently massaged on the tip of penis (i.e. is entire glans penis), and message till the fluid is fully absorbed by the glans penis. If it is' applied judiciously and cautiously, you can enjoy added joy from coitus and also you won't ejaculate, early.

Important Yogic Exercises for Better Sex Life

For prolongation of sexual union, and the ecstasy, the following asanas and bandhas are of special interest :-

1. Padmasana
2. Siddhasana
3. Baddha Konasana
4. Vajrasana
5. Chakrasana
6. Uddiyanabandha
7. Mula Bandha
8. Shavasana

Padmasana or the Lotus pose

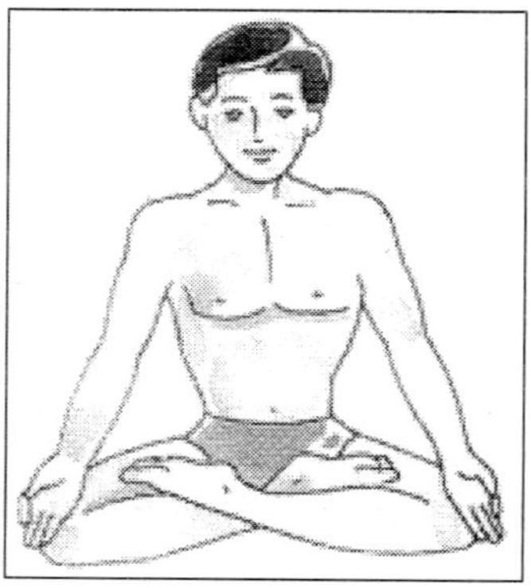

The Lotus pose is a basic and versatile pose symbolizing man's spiritual growth, evolution, purity and peace. Padma means lotus. It is called padmasana because it is in imitation of lotus more in nature than in appearance. This posture is classic for meditation and pranayam. Lord Budha and other great yogis are generally shown sitting in this pose.

Technique -

1. Sit erect on the floor with both your legs stretched in front.
2. Bend the right knee folding the leg and put the foot high on left thigh.
3. Bring the left foot similarly and place it high on the right thigh.
4. Both the knees should touch the ground and keep both the heels near navel. Keep the soles of the feet up turned.
5. Spread out the arms and place the palms on the knees. Make a loop of the index finger and the thumb by touching each other. Keep other fingers joined and stretched.
6. Change the legs after some time. Now, keep the left leg first and then the right leg. It helps in developing the legs evenly.
7. In the beginning you may feel pain in your knees and ankles, but practice makes it comfortable even for longer sessions.

Effects

1. In this posture pelvis gets richer blood supply and tones up coccygeal and sacral nerves.
2. It keeps the mind alert and steady and ankles and knees supple.
3. For pranayama it is the best and the mind grows calm and clear.
4. The erect spine makes one's concentration strong and lasting. It helps in the awakening of Kundalini as it can be maintained for hours at a stretch without any discomfort.
5. This pose also helps in removing constipation. During this meditative pose the production of carbon dioxide is reduced to the minimum.

Siddhasana or the accomplished pose

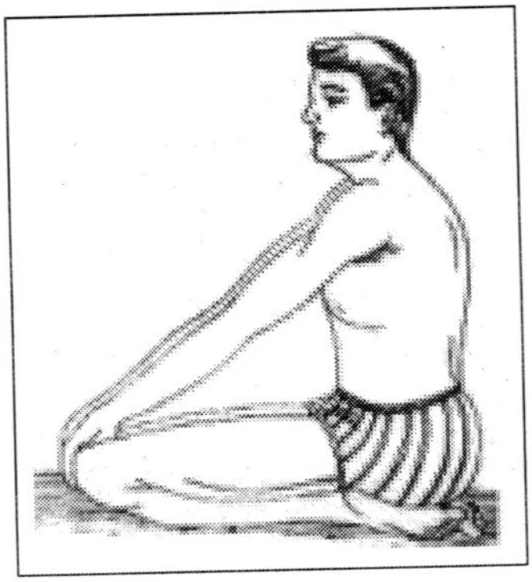

Siddha means an adept or an accomplished person. This posture is favourite of accomplished yogis, hence this name.

Technique

1. Sit down on the floor with legs out stretched in front. Bend the left leg at the knee and fold it so as the heel sets tightly against your perinium for this purpose hold up your genitals with the left hand.
2. Keep the sole of the left foot touching the right thigh and the pressure of the heel on both sides of perineum.
3. Rest your genitals between the left thigh and left calf.
4. Now fold in the left leg so as its heel is placed above the penis near the pubic bones. The right sole rests between the thigh and the calf of the left leg.
5. Stretch the arms in front with the back of the palms resting on the knees. Join the thumbs and the index fingers into rings. Rest of the fingers remain together and stretched. This is known as Gyana mudra.
6. Keep the head, neck and the back erect and in a line, Remain in the pose as long as possible, come out of the pose, relax a little and repeat changing the order of legs.

Effects

1. Like Padamasana, Sidhasana is a classic and basic pose. It relaxes the whole body while keeping one alert and watchful.
2. This pose is good for pranayam and Meditation as is Padamasana.
3. It makes the movement of ankles and knees smooth and stimulates abdominal region.

sitting in this pose.

Technique -

1. Sit erect on the floor with both your legs stretched in front.
2. Bend the right knee folding the leg and put the foot high on left thigh.
3. Bring the left foot similarly and place it high on the right thigh.
4. Both the knees should touch the ground and keep both the heels near navel. Keep the soles of the feet up turned.
5. Spread out the arms and place the palms on the knees. Make a loop of the index finger and the thumb by touching each other. Keep other fingers joined and stretched.
6. Change the legs after some time. Now, keep the left leg first and then the right leg. It helps in developing the legs evenly.
7. In the beginning you may feel pain in your knees and ankles, but practice makes it comfortable even for longer sessions.

Effects

1. In this posture pelvis gets richer blood supply and tones up coccygeal and sacral nerves.
2. It keeps the mind alert and steady and ankles and knees supple.
3. For pranayama it is the best and the mind grows calm and clear.
4. The erect spine makes one's concentration strong and lasting. It helps in the awakening of Kundalini as it can be maintained for hours at a stretch without any discomfort.
5. This pose also helps in removing constipation. During this meditative pose the production of carbon dioxide is reduced to the minimum.

Siddhasana or the accomplished pose

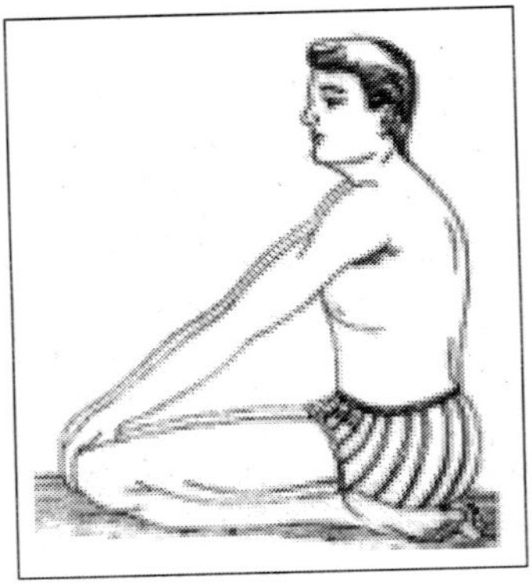

Siddha means an adept or an accomplished person. This posture is favourite of accomplished yogis, hence this name.

Technique

1. Sit down on the floor with legs out stretched in front. Bend the left leg at the knee and fold it so as the heel sets tightly against your perinium for this purpose hold up your genitals with the left hand.
2. Keep the sole of the left foot touching the right thigh and the pressure of the heel on both sides of perineum.
3. Rest your genitals between the left thigh and left calf.
4. Now fold in the left leg so as its heel is placed above the penis near the pubic bones. The right sole rests between the thigh and the calf of the left leg.
5. Stretch the arms in front with the back of the palms resting on the knees. Join the thumbs and the index fingers into rings. Rest of the fingers remain together and stretched. This is known as Gyana mudra.
6. Keep the head, neck and the back erect and in a line, Remain in the pose as long as possible, come out of the pose, relax a little and repeat changing the order of legs.

Effects

1. Like Padamasana, Sidhasana is a classic and basic pose. It relaxes the whole body while keeping one alert and watchful.
2. This pose is good for pranayam and Meditation as is Padamasana.
3. It makes the movement of ankles and knees smooth and stimulates abdominal region.

Baddha Konasana

Technique

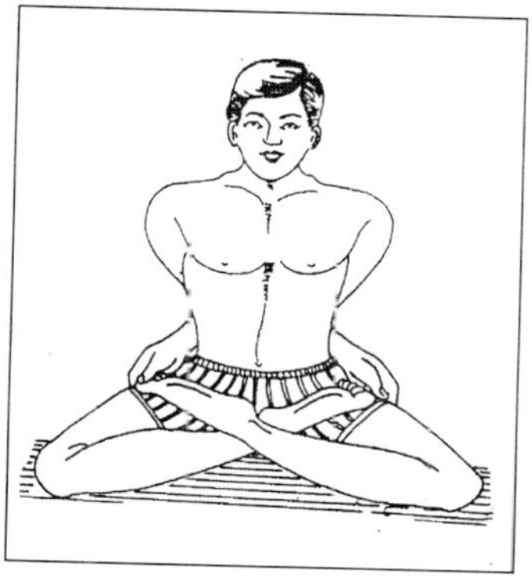

1. Sit down on the floor with the legs stretched and together in front.
2. Rest the palms on the floor in your sides, the fingers pointing.
3. Keeping the back erect end both the legs at knees and fold in by catching the feet with both the hands. Draw the heels near your perinium. The sole of both the feet should remain joined.
4. Pressing the thighs with your elbows make them touch the floor. Keep the thighs wide also. Remain in the pose for 30 seconds with normal breathing and than release the feet and relax.

Effects

1. It is to benefit much those with urinary troubles, the abdominal region, back and prevails are invigorated as a result of richer blood supply.
2. It keeps the kidneys and the prostate in good health.
3. It is very good for patients of hernia. It relieves sciatic pain and heaviness of testicles. Removes seminal weakness.
4. It's very beneficial for women as regards menstrual disorders etc.
5. It's daily practice helps a pregnant woman in delivery the baby easily.
6. It can be practised even after meals.

Vajrasana or the Hardy Pose

Technique

1. Kneel down on the floor with your knees, ankles and big tocs touching the ground.

2. Sit down on your heels and place your palms on the knees.
3. Keep yourself erect but relaxed. Breathe deeply and slowly.
4. Expand your chest and the abdominal region inward.

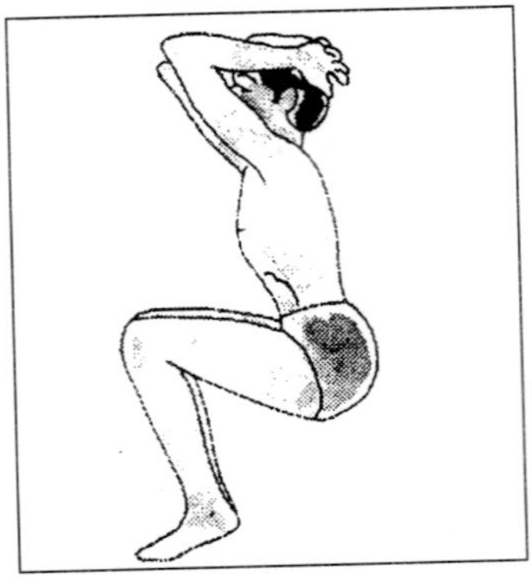

Effects

1. It is good for people suffering from blood pressure.
2. It can be practised any time even after taking meals.
3. It strengthens spine, removes pain in spine and tones up sexual organs both in male and female.
4. Gives longevity and postpones old age.

Chakrasana or the wheel pose :

In this pose the body assumes the shape of a wheel hence this name Chakra means a wheel.

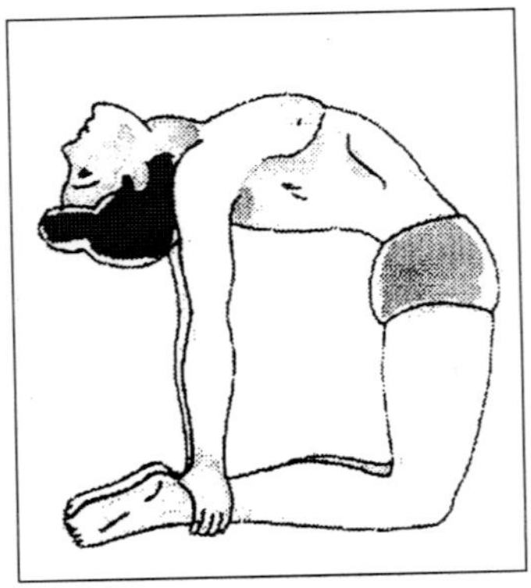

Technique

1. Lie down on your back on the floor flat, bend your knees, your heels touching your buttocks.
2. Fold the arms backwards at elbows with palms under the shoulders resting on the ground and fingers pointing towards your trunk.
3. Keep the arms and the legs apart, inhale, raise your hips and pressing the palms on the floor gently, rest the top of your head on the floor pause for a few moments.
4. Inhale and raise your head straightening your hands, raise your hips higher.

5. Try to bring the feet closer to the pals till they touch one another, but do not strain. Take your own time in achieving it.
6. Keep normal but deep breathing during the holding of the posture. Maintain firm hold on the ground with your feet and the palms.
7. Reverse the steps and come down slowly to the floor and relax.

Uddiyana Bandha

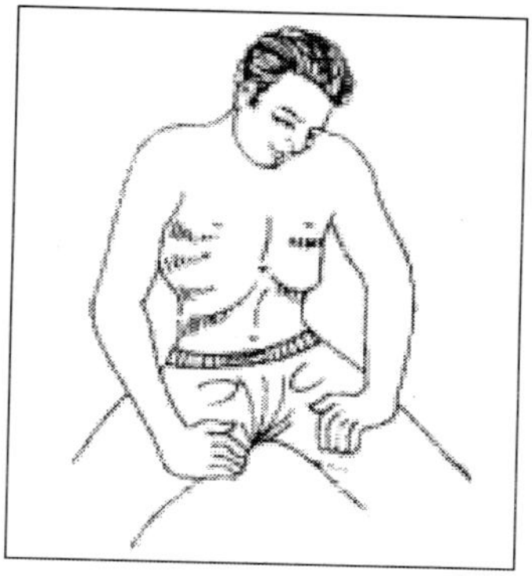

It is very powerful bandha and a basic one for regulating the flow of prana and awakening of kundalini. Uddiyana involves the lifting up of the Diaphragm high up the chest and pulling up the abdominal organs towards the spine. It means to fly up. This bandha marks the great bird of prana fly towards the highest chakra Brhmrandhra or Sahasraara. It is to be practised between the full exhalation and fresh inhalation. When the breath is suspended. Once in a day, early in the morning it should be practised, first standing, then, in advanced stage, in sitting position.

Bandha literally means a lock, bondage, joining together, etc. In a bandha certain organs and parts of the body are controlled and contracted. Bandhas are necessary to prevent the dissipation of pranic energy and its proper and maximum utilization. A bandha is a special posture invented to conserve and make a greater use of vast resources of energy, generated by yogic exercises and pranayam. Bandhas should be practised separately in the beginning, before they are incorporated in pranayam.

During yoga the prana is made to flow in attendance through the nervous system and helps in carrying this extra energy of prana to the right organ without causing harm to any other part of the organism. Without proper channelisation of prana, it may prove lethal. Thus bandhas are a means of reorientation and control of pranic energy.

Technique

1. Stand erect on your feet one foot apart.
2. Bend the knees a little and then slightly bend forward.
3. Rest palms, with fingers spread, on your thighs above the knees.
4. Take a few deep breaths and then exhale forcefully so as to empty your lungs completely. Press your chin against the chest in chin lock.
5. Keep the breath suspended and pull the entire abdominal region back towards your spine. Then draw it up towards thorax, keep the pressure of your palms on the thighs all this time. Remain in the posse for 20-30 seconds according to your capacity.
6. Relax the grip on your abdominal region and inhale slowly and deeply.
7. Repeat the cycle 3-5 times.

Effects

1. Uddiyana Bandha is of great spiritual value as it forces the prana up the Sushuma nadi.
2. It invigorates the whole abdominal region.
3. It rejuvenates an old person, if it is properly and constantly practised.
4. The uplifting of diaphragm massages the heart muscles.

Mula Bandha

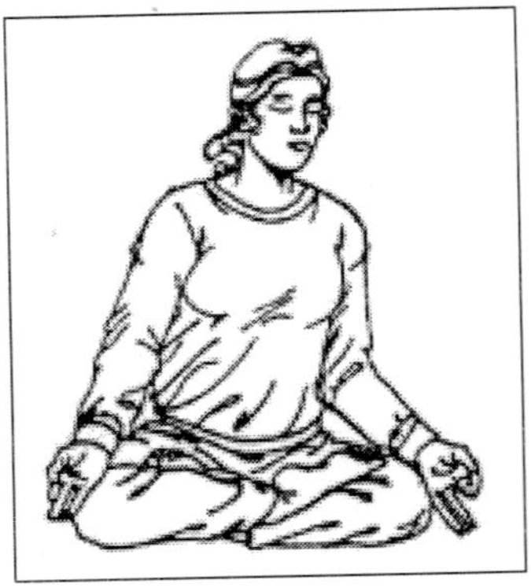

Mula literally means the root, source, foundation or the basis. In it, the portion between anus and scrotum is contracted and raised. This prevents apaana escaping from the lower body and draws it up to unite with prana.

Technique

1. Sit in Padmasana or Siddhasana. Stretch your hands and fingers in Gyana Mudra.
2. Inhale deeply and retain it. Press the chin against the chest in chin lock.
3. Contract the region of lower abdomen between the anus and the navel towards your spine and pull it up towards the diaphragm.
4. Now, contract and pull upwards the abdominal muscles and remain in the posture for a few seconds.
5. Release the grip and sphinec and abdominal muscles, remove the chin lock. Exhale slowly and evenly. Repeat the cycle 3-5 times.

Effects

1. It prevents apaana escaping from the lower body and draws it up to unite with prana.
2. It increases sexual retention power and gives a person of great moral and spiritual power.
3. It helps much in awakening the dormant Kundalini by preventing the dissipation of pranic energy and changing it into a physical force.
4. Mula Bandha may be practised later on, in advanced stage in doing shirasana, sarvangasana, paschimottanasana, etc.

It is beyond any shadow of doubt that Hatha Yoga, increases the sex power. and Hatha Yoga, makes sex sacramental by elevating it to the great spiritual level and heights. The prolonged ecstasy obtained through sexo-yogic postures is to be practised regularly. Our great ancient yogis, sages and seers have recommended the judicious blending of sex and yoga to experience the divine ecstasy and rapport leading to samadhi. There is no sex stimulant or aphrodisiac as efficacious and regarding as the Yogasanas. The peak experience of orgasm arising out of such a union cannot be defined in words.

Shavasana or the Corpse pose

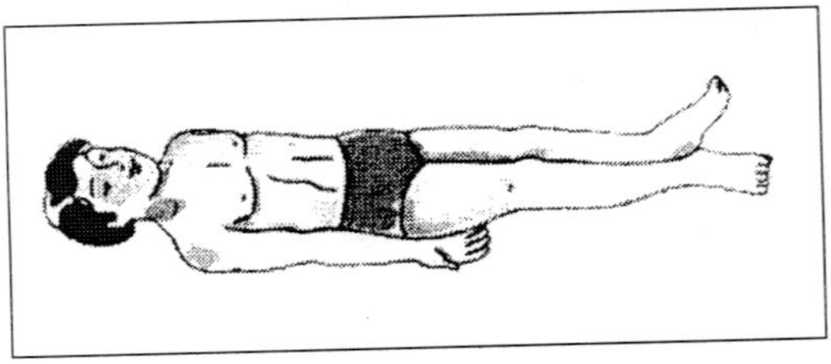

This classic, simple, yet difficult, posture is to be practised before and after the each session and in between the various asanas. This pose is called shavasana or the Corpse Pose because it imitates a dead body or a corpse and provides relaxation to the muscles and mind. Shava means a dead body.

Technique

1. Lie down flat on your back like a corpse.
2. Keep the hands at a little distance from the thighs and the palms up.
3. Let the feet be apart at 1½ feet distance and the eyes closed.
4. Take a long deep breath and then breathe slowly, and rhythmically so as not to disturb your body. Inhalataion and exhalation should be equal and uniform. There should be no effort to increase the volume of respiration . Arythmical breathing is all that is most required.
5. Concentrate on your respiration and relax completely. Keep the jaws loose and not clenched. Let there be no movement either of the pupils or the tongue.
6. In the beginning you may fall asleep but when by practice you immerse into deep relaxation, you would feel your body and mind grown still, detached and completely relaxed.
7. Autosuggestion is wonderful here, Repeat in your mind' I relax the feet, they are relaxed. I relax the legs, they are relaxed, "Then take your abdomen, chest and hands one by one. The hand and brain may come up the last. Thus bring all the parts of your body

under relaxation simultaneously.

8. In the end of a session, of asanas. It should be practised for ten minutes and in between various asanas for three minutes.

Effects

1. It removes fatigue caused by other asanas and induces calmness of mind. It makes one feel one's mind like a deep, still, clear pool of water, without ripple. Dive deep into this pool and emerge refreshed and relaxed.
2. Steady, smooth, uniforms and fine respiration soothes the nerves, muscles and calms the brain.
3. It reduces high blood pressure, tension, and fatigue, The whole nervous system is toned up resulting in increased concentration.
4. In these times of strain and stress there cannot be any better antidote than Shavasana. It should be practised as many times a day as possible.

Indians Lose Virginity at the Average Age of 19.8

India, is changing. A society where the word sex was once considered a taboo, it is now increasingly talking about sex education and AIDS awareness. This is just one of the many suprising findings that the Durex Global Sex Survey 2005—cutting across 41 countries and questioning 3,17,000 respondents—has come up with. However, awareness must not be confused with embracing the Western values completely. Indians still frown at both extramarital and pre-marital sex. They have the fewest sexual partners (three, compared to the Turkish number of 14.5). Only 13 per cent Indians have a one-night stand and they are among the oldest to lose their virginity at 19.8 years!

For all those who have been talking about marriage meeting its nemesis in the Indian metros, here's a befitting reply: About 46 per cent Indians are happy with their sex lives as compared to 44 per cent people worldwide.

Indians are also among the most aware when it comes to the HIV/AIDS menace and unsafe sex: While 87 per cent Indians feel HIV/AIDS is a top priority area, only 72 per cent people globly think so. Their mantra is 'play safe' when it comess to unprotected sex, and only 21 per cent Indians have indulged in such behaviour.

The importance of sex education is increasingly being realised in the country and people feel that it should begin by age 14. For a conservative society, India is making significant strides when it comes to AIDS awareness and sex education, but is this enough?

Is India aware of the AIDS menace?

India is in the grip of AIDS manace: There area about 5.1 million HIV+ patients and 1,11,608 people with AIDS in India. However, it's interesting to note that over 87 per cent of Indians believe that HIV/AIDS is the most important area that needs greater public awareness, while only 72 per cent of people globally felt so. So, is India finally waking up to the AIDS menace?

What is the right age for sex education?

Sex education, till now, has been a red herring for both Indian schools and parents. The situation is gradually changing, with 14 now considered the right age for children to get sex education as compared to 15.6 years earlier. However, it falls way short of global average, which says that sex education should begin by 12 years. With the 15-25 age-group being worst affected by AIDS in India, is 14 early enough?

Is India still conservative?

Despite what society watchers will make you believe, India's morals have not changed. We still remain one of the most conservative societies worldwide. According to the survey, close to half the respondents (49 per cent) feel young people should abstain from pre-marital sex. We are also at the bottom of the rung when it comes to extra-marital affairs (15 per cent) compared to 22 per cent globally.

What is the age for first-time sex?

Indians are the oldest to lose their virginity. And the average age for the young adults here is 19.8 years as against 17.3 years which has been cited as the average age of first-time sex for people in other parts of the world. Guess which country starts out fairly early in this regard? Compared to other countries, it's Iceland where people have sex as early as 15.6 years. Germany with its age of 15.9 years and Sweden with 16.1 years follow close behind.

Who should impart sex education?

Whose responsibility is it anyway? Should schools be the one imparting sex education or should the onus fall on parents? The debate continues.... According to the survey, parents accept sex education is important but want the schools to take the onus. So, while 47 per cent Indians think government should invest more in schools to make sex education available to students at an early age, only 34 per cent people around the world think so.

......What it means

Film director Revathi, who did extensive research on the subject, feels that while films like hers do reach out to the urban crowd, the rural areas still need to be tapped. "The campaigns must highlight the importance of protected sex and the need for sticking to one partner. The only way out is to talk – for, the more we talk, the more awareness we spread."

Says Jitender Nagpal, psychologist, who is involved in drafting of the NCERT's National Curriculum Framework, "We need to provide an integrated, age-specific sex education to children. If they are denied the right knowledge, they would only fall back on other sources which will be either concocted or inadequate. And going by the AIDS figures in India, we just cannot afford doing this."

Says Shobha De, author, "Sex has always been a taboo subject, even for this generation of parents and kids. It's still a forbidden territory in India. As far as youngers are concerned, sex and responsibility go together. you have to be emotionally mature to deal with your sexual attitudes. So, our society is conservative, but in a realistic way."

"Why must a big deal be made about virginity," asks

Anita Roy, commissioning editor for *Young Zubaan* books for young adults and children. "The age for lossing virginity is irrelevent. What is relevent is what they lose and gain out of it," she says. She would cite the age of losing virginity as much older than 19.8 years, despite "the media talking about how fast society is moving towards promiscuity."

Most parents in India are not aware of their role in imparting sex education. Says Amit Jain, sex counsellor, "sex education doesn't even figure at all in the priorities of the Indian parents. Instead of blamming schools, they should understand that it's a partnership between parents and the schools." Adds Nagpal, "It is always the parents to whom a child will go first when such questions come to his mind, rest of the sources are a distant second."

–

Courtesy - *TOI*

Other Books on

HEALTH SERIES

1. Yog Chikitsa (Hindi) **(New)** 295/-
2. Yoga for Health and Relaxation **(New)** 160/-
3. Yoga for All **(New)** 295/-
4. Yoga for Daily Life **(New)** 350/-
5. Complete Book of Yoga **(New)** 195/-
6. Yoga Therapy **(New)** 275/-
7. A Guide to Your Pregnancy **(New)** 195/-
8. Ayurveda for All 195/-
9. A Guide to Migraine, Airthritis, Cervical Spondylosis, and Backache 150/-
10. Body and Beauty Care 150/-
11. Child Care and Nutrition 175/-
12. Naturopathy Modern Way of Life 195/-
13. First Aid How to Handle an Accident 125/-
14. Acupressure in Daily Life 195/-
15. Look Younger at Any Age 195/-
16. HIV/AIDS - Transmission, Prevention and A. Therapies125/-
17. Diabetics and Diet 195/-
18. Increase your Height & Loose your Weight 195/-
19. Make Fitness A Way of Life 195/-
20. Common Problems of Children 225/-
21. Handbook of Nutrition & Dietetics 295/-
22. A Guide to Massage Therapy 195/-
23. A Guide to Family Medicine 150/-
24. A Guide to Digestive Disorders 195/-
25. Complete Book of Child Care 160/-
26. A Guide to Homoeopathy 195/-
27. Life Begins at 40 195/-
28. Alternative Therapies 150/-
29. How to Overcome Stress 195/-
30. Obesity 225/-
31. Self Motivation 175/-
32. Women Disorders and Pregnancy 125/-
33. A Guide to Body Pains 160/-
34. Sex Education 195/-
35. Common Diseases and Cure 195/-
36. Pranayama for Better Life 195/-
37. Herbal Home Remedies 195/-
38. A Guide to Beauty & Skin Care 195/-
39. A Guide to Heart Care 195/-
40. A Guide to High Blood Pressure 195/-
41. Cancer Causes and Prevention 250/-
42. Nature Cure for Common Diseases 150/-
43. Good Health Through Food and Regimen 110/-
44. A Guide to Allergies 225/-
45. A Guide to Aging 175/-
46. Ayurveda for Health & Beauty 175/-